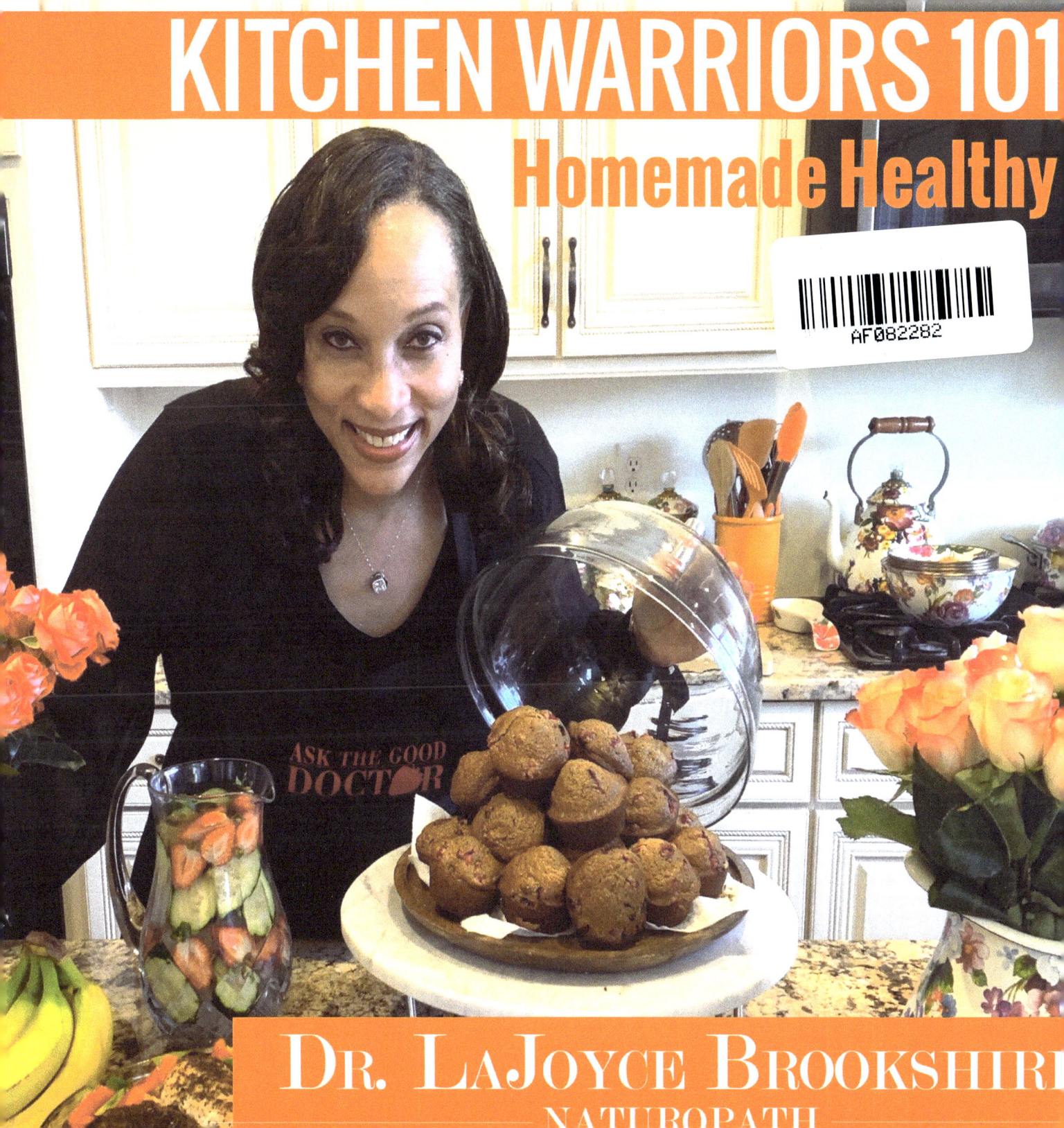

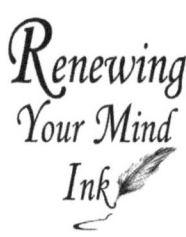

Copyright 2020 © Dr. LaJoyce Brookshire

The following photos are credited to Irvin Wright:
Pineapple Upside Cake (p. 145), apron (p. 154), back cover.

PUBLISHER'S NOTE:
Printed and bound in the United States of America. All rights reserved.
No part of this book may be reproduced or transmitted in any form or by any means, electronic or mechanical, including photocopying, recording, or by any information storage and retrieval system except by a reviewer who may quote brief passages in a review to be printed in a magazine, newspaper, or on the Web without permission in writing from the publisher.

Ordering Information: Quantity sales. Special discounts are available on quantity purchases by corporations, associations, and others. For details, contact the publisher at the address below.

Although the author and publisher have made every effort to ensure the accuracy and completeness of information contained in this book, we assume no responsibility for errors, inaccuracies, omissions, or any inconsistency herein.

ISBN: 978-1-58441-003-4

Renewing Your Mind Ink and Peace in the Storm Publishing, LLC.
Visit our Website at www.peaceinthestormpublishing.com

This book is lovingly dedicated to my mother, Joana Hunter Baker, who taught me the importance of cooking fresh food daily; my husband, Gus, and daughter, Brooke, who eat all I put before them; and in memory of my Grannie Fannie, Aunt Nita, and Aunt Mabel who walked me through more recipes than I can ever find the space to write, and who gave me enough china, silver, and utensils for a lifetime…

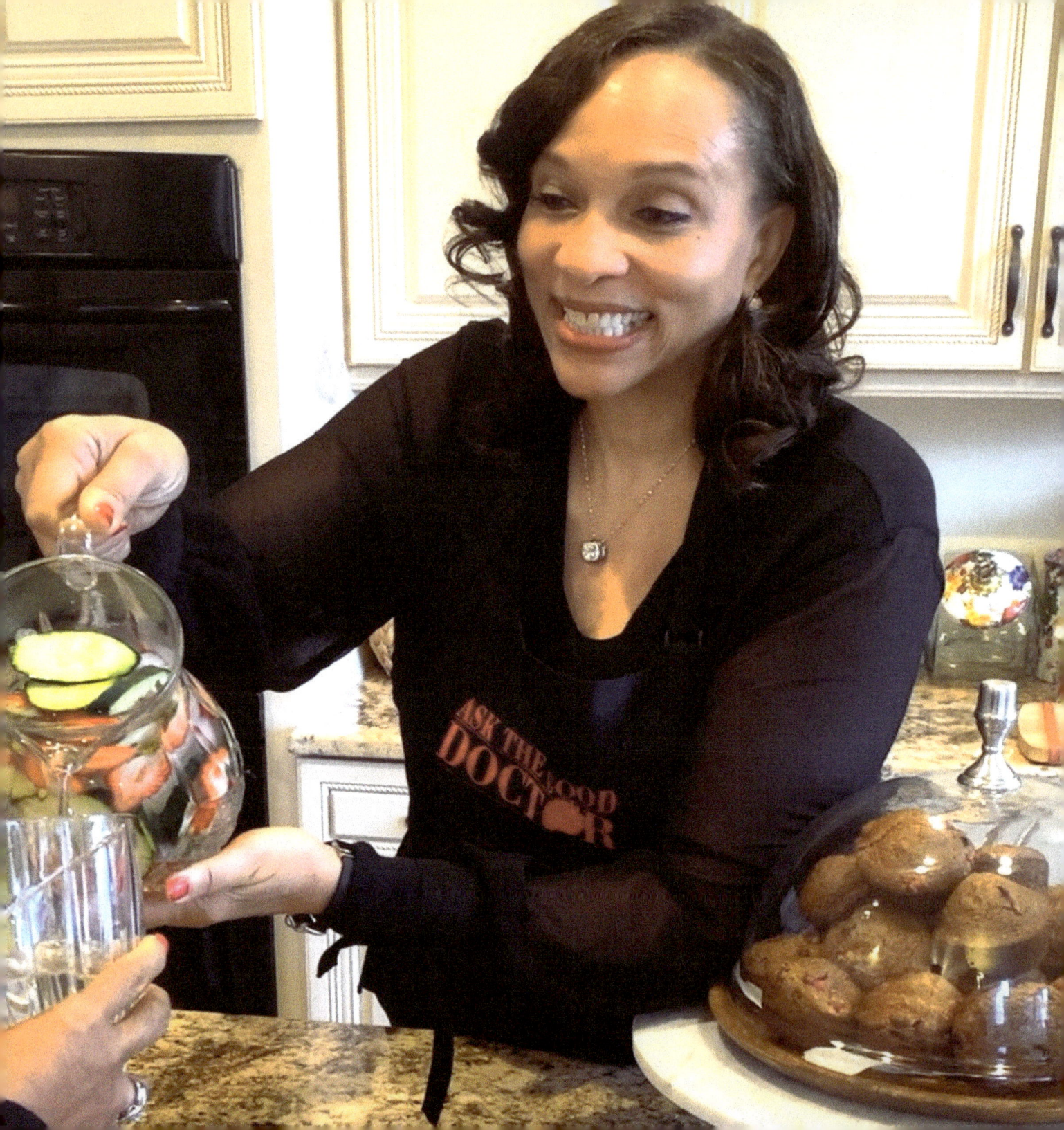

Dr. LaJoyce Brookshire, a Classical Naturopathic Doctor and Host of the SiriusXM UrbanView Show, ASK THE GOOD DOCTOR, is committed to teaching how to Attain, Maintain, and Reclaim Perfect Health. She is an advocate for farm fresh organic ingredients to make delicious food. Homemade Healthy is a remix of many comfort foods, swapping unhealthy ingredients for healthy alternatives. Included is a shopping list, Nutritional Notes, and anecdotes.

Dr.Brookshire believes that "our biography does not dictate our biology and what we inherit is not disease but recipes." Since she was a young girl, Dr. Brookshire has had a fascination with cooking. Hailing from a long line of professional chefs, she has been a KITCHEN WARRIOR, remixing recipes from her Easy Bake Oven to World Class Kitchens at Culinary Resorts. Today, Dr. Brookshire spins traditional favorites into nutritional dishes worthy of *Mmmmmmm* with every bite.

Health is determined by what's on your plate and not what is in a bag, a box, or drive-thru. Become a KITCHEN WARRIOR and Make it Yourself... Make it Fresh... Make it Homemade Healthy.

Contents

Introduction	1
How to Shop	5
In the Cabinet	12
Recipes	16
Beverages	19
Breakfast	32
Lunch	42
Vegetables	51
Snacks, Salads, & Appetizers	67
Soups	83
Entrées	96
Sides	124
Desserts	136

Introduction

It was 1979 when I was a senior in high school that I first began my Wellness Journey. Thanks to Cyndi Rodgers who gave a Persuasive Speech in our honors English class about why you should not eat meat. The speech was riveting! Cyndi had visual aids to show the body systems of those who eat meat and those who did not. I was sold by the time she explained the brain function of a child who had never eaten meat versus the child who had always been a carnivorous consumer.

I was so persuaded to try her suggestions that when I left class, I went to the lunch room and ordered a grilled cheese sandwich on rye. That night I announced to my mother, "I am never eating meat again! I'm a vegetarian."

She unenthusiastically responded, "Help yourself, there's some salad in the refrigerator," thinking it was just another one of my phases.

A few weeks later I landed a job at General Nutrition Center (GNC) in Evergreen Plaza in Chicago. In 1979, GNC was the Whole Foods of our day. Back then, GNC actually sold groceries, juiced juices, ground peanut butter, and had sandwiches. I learned a wealth of information and I was even more sold out to my new lifestyle.

By the time I went to Eastern Illinois University in the fall of 1980 I was armed with boxes of herbs, vitamin supplements, and information. I quickly became known by my friends as the go-to-girl who could whip up a little something and make you feel better. My vegetarian lifestyle only lasted until Christmas of my freshman year because my hair started falling out as it was very difficult for me to adequately replace my proteins. I had completely lost the taste for beef and pork so I slowly began re-introducing chicken, turkey, and fish. Gratefully after about a month my hair stopped falling out and it caused me to take a closer look at exactly what I was eating. I found it very interesting that with just the addition of one meat protein daily there was a big difference. At seventeen years old I was not that good of a cook and with my living in an off-campus apartment I was handicapped when it came to making protein varieties. One thing was for sure…because of my GNC "education" I was never going to go back to eating all of the crap I used to eat.

Other good lifestyle habits that I possessed were going to bed early, getting up early, and getting exercise. I had all eight o'clock classes in college and would be finished daily by noon. I had time to study, work, and yes, even party all by ten o'clock when I would absolutely be in bed! I have always been the sleepyhead in my crew and all of my friends have photos of me asleep at a party somewhere. The body only heals when we are sleeping during the night so sleep is VERY important.

Upon college graduation at age 21, I entered my field of study in broadcast journalism and moved to New York City. Not long after the move I noticed the need to up the intake of my supplements due to the nature of big city stressors. With millions of people come millions of more germs, many more opportunities to socialize and party, more stress at work, and yes, the stress of getting *to* work on the beloved subway system. My body had taken a beating that only I knew I was experiencing—constipation, acrid urine, body aches, and intermittent facial breakouts all of which were foreign to me. It was an interesting observation to me that my peers were always complimenting my clear skin. Aren't all twenty-two year olds straight-out-of-college supposed to be bright-eyed, fresh-faced, and over-joyed with the smell of success that New York City opportunities can bring? Instead I was surrounded with what should have been vibrant twenty-somethings who had allowed New York to chew them up and spit them out. This was the fuel I needed to become what some called a "Health Nut". I did not care not one bit about the names I was being called. I was healthy and in love with the life and the knowledge God had blessed me to have.

In 1990, I fell in love with Prince Charming and we were married within the year. He was so critical of my healthy eating habits that he and his family called me Rabbit. To this day I have never seen one family consume so much meat and so many fast food meals! Two years into our marriage, I found out that my Prince married me knowing he had AIDS and never told me. After one year of dating, two years of marriage, and lots of unprotected sex, it's funny…he never mentioned it. The blessing in it all is that I am still alive AND HIV negative! Many say I am a miracle walking. My response is simply that I am God's Girl. I believe in Jesus Christ and I am convinced about the miraculous power of protection His blood offers those who are His children. (Read the full account of this story in *Faith under Fire: Betrayed by a Thing Called Love* on Karen Hunter Publishing/Pocket Books/Simon Schuster).

I also have to give credit to the rock solid immune system I have acquired as a result of the healthy lifestyle I had been following for the last ten years *before* that situation. I am a living, breathing, real life example of how when your immune system is strong, you can be exposed to ANYthing and you will not become affected. Dr. Joseph Mercola says:

> *"It is my belief, and that of nearly all natural health care practitioners, that these infectious agents only serve as triggers to cause the illness, but what is required or responsible for the actual infection is a dysfunctional immune system. I use the analogy of disease to darkness and health to light. If you shine a light in a dark room it is not dark anymore. Darkness and light simply can't coexist. Similarly if you are*

healthy you can have massive exposure to infectious agents and you simply will NOT get sick. Just like light and darkness it is very difficult, if not impossible in most cases, for a strong immune system and infectious disease to exist together. It is the state of your immune system—not the bacteria or virus itself—that determines whether or not you will get sick, even if you come in contact with the germ."

To that, I say…Amen!

In 2001 I entered the doctorate program at Trinity College of Natural Health to become a Classical Doctor of Naturopathy, Master Herbalist, and Doctor of Naturopathic Ministry so that I could attach some credibility to all of the "unofficial" good advice I had been dishing out to my family and friends.

A Classical Naturopathic Doctor treats with everything that is in nature to help keep you well. It is necessary to tackle sickness and disease with holistic approaches starting with building and maintaining the immune system and proper levels of acidity. When you give the body what it needs, it *will* repair itself. To some this simple premise seems, well...too simple. To others it seems quite logical. I thrive on teaching the principles to uncomplicate the premise of staying well to those who have complicated the issue. As a result of these teachings, my former student, Karu Daniels has affectionately called me The *Good* Doctor for many years. It is how I have arrived at the description of myself and the work that I desire to continue for the rest of my days on earth.

In the first book of the *Ask The Good Doctor* series *The Detox Edition* (available as an e-book at Amazon.com), I teach seven easy steps to the detoxification process. This recipe book will aid with meals for detoxing and for every day enjoyment. On these pages it is my hope you will come to understand that there are catalysts which trigger positive and negative responses in our bodies. One catalyst is food; the other catalyst is emotion. The next great weapons for maintaining good health are your foods and your thoughts. Food and thoughts can usher in cancer or combat cancer. Food and thoughts can lead you into diabetes or lead you out of a diabetic state. The adage that states You Are What You Eat should be accompanied by "*You are what you think.*" For the Bible says in Proverbs 23:7, "*As a man thinketh in his heart so is he.*"

Read on and learn…

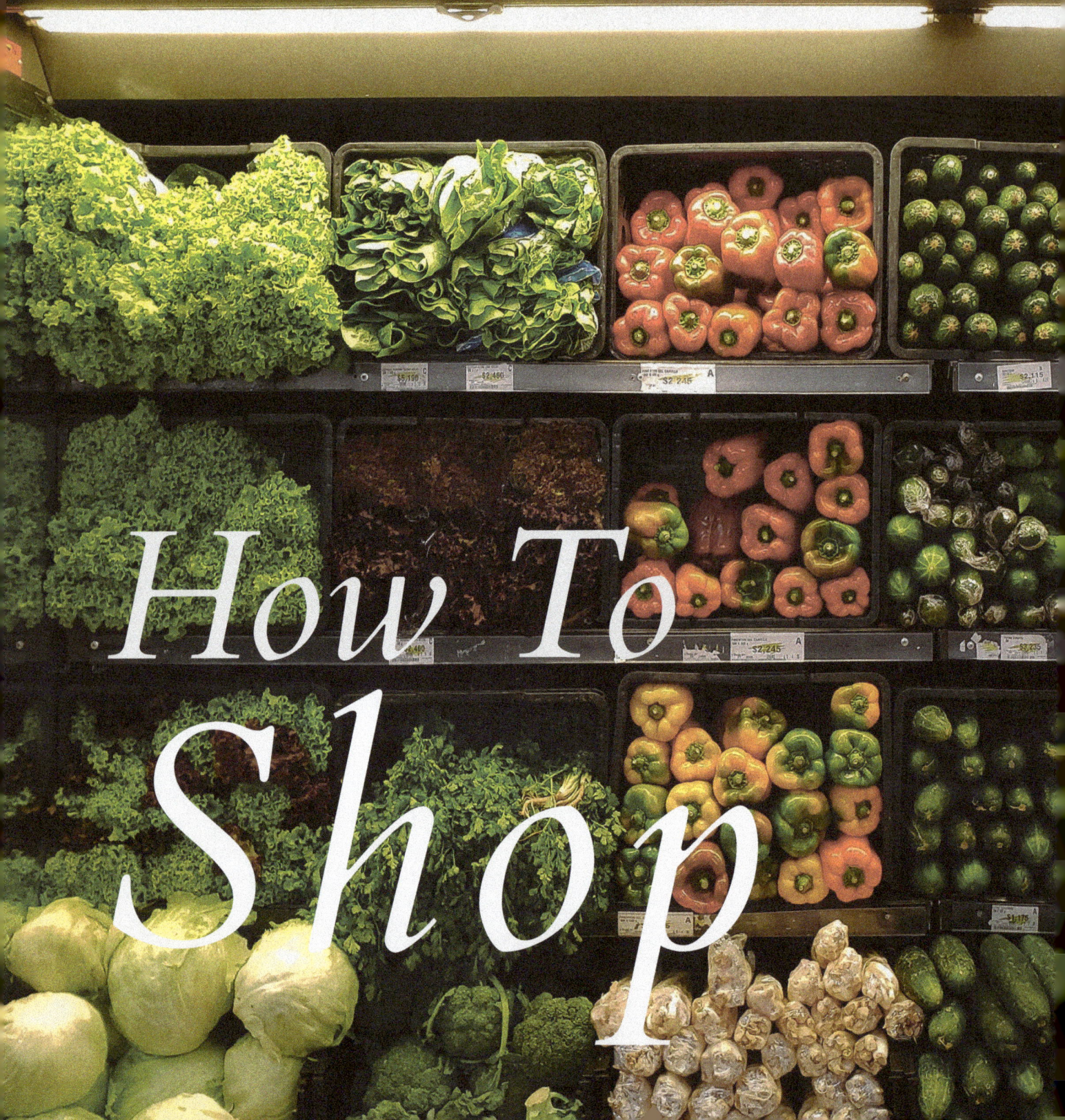

Grocery shopping should be an absolute joy. Many on the quest for better health practices and a better lifestyle blame the expense as to why they are not compliant. Just as we bargain shop for dresses and shoes, so must we for healthy food. I begin with the sales papers and scour for organic products on sale. From May through October I delight in the local Farmer's Market and buy fresh produce from local and organic farms.

The Farmer's Market adventure should begin with what looks freshest and the most delicious. When confronted with a vegetable or fruit that is unfamiliar to you, don't hesitate to ask the farmer, "How is this best prepared?" Often-times there are samples readily available. One of my favorite obscure finds is Garlic Scape, which is the coarse, green, curly, stem that first sprouts out of the ground just ahead of the garlic bulbs. The flavor is intensely garlicky and pungent. I mince the Scape in a food processor, portion into freezer bags, and into ice cube trays. The ice cubed version is very handy when making soups and beans. The freezer bagged Scape can be sautéed for omelets, stir-fry, or for a fresh dip with sour cream.

The Beekeeper—Local raw honey is also the absolute best for your health and to taste. We should always consume honey that is harvested within 100 miles of where you live because your body is familiar with the local pollen and allergic reactions would be minimal.

The Dairy Man—The trip would not be complete without a stop by the local dairy stand for farm fresh eggs, unpasteurized raw milk directly

goodness of others. Fresh baked bread with hearty multi-grains, sprouts, and herbs are so aromatic that it cannot be resisted. I never leave the market without a square of buttermilk crumb cake topped with raspberry, blackberry or blueberry goodness.

On Saturday mornings, my daughter Brooke and I leave the house hungry and eat our way across the Farmer's Market enjoying the freshness of the foods and knowing we have supported the local farmer.

Newsflash—No farms, No food. Isn't that an intense concept to grasp? But we can each do our share by changing our buying patterns. There are a lot of grocery store chains who buy produce from local farms and they proudly display signs to advise the conscious consumer.

Many abort their commitment to a healthy lifestyle because of the expense. And yes, the stuff that has the most dirt on it costs the most. The best way to survive the decision to maintain your lifestyle change to keep you well is to scour the sales circulars for the best prices starting with organic items and then No Antibiotic/No Hormone/No GMO's (Genetically Modified Organisms) products. Beware of the companies we grew up with who have now jumped on the "organic" bandwagon since it has become a multi-billion-dollar industry. I will not buy an organic Keebler cracker nor an organic Tyson Chicken. I will continue to support the companies who have a history of feeding well us without poison.

Armed with the circulars to help save you money, the grocery store adventure should begin in the produce section. Fresh fruits and vegetables should be atop of the list. We know it is best to purchase organics due to the amount of pesticides that are on the food. The argument to purchase organic sometimes goes out the window due to the expense. The Environmental Working Group (EWG) is an organization dedicated to creating a list it calls the *Dirty Dozen* which names the worst offenders. It is really smart shopping to be able to arm yourself with information in an effort to decrease exposures to pesticides.

The 12 most contaminated fruits and veggies are when you should look for a sale and <u>always</u> buy organic according to EWG's **Dirty Dozen**:

1. Celery
2. Peaches
3. Strawberries
4. Apples
5. Blueberries
6. Nectarines
7. Bell Peppers
8. Spinach
9. Kale
10. Cherries
11. Potatoes
12. Imported Grapes

EWG also has a list called **The Clean Fifteen**. This list touts the cleanest conventional fruits and vegetables to buy.

When the Farmer's Market is in season, the grocery store should be a supplement. Weekly fresh items from the peripheral isles of the store should include:

1. Onions
2. Avocado
3. Sweet Corn
4. Pineapple
5. Mangos
6. Sweet Peas
7. Asparagus
8. Kiwi
9. Cabbage
10. Eggplant
11. Cantaloupe
12. Watermelon
13. Grapefruit
14. Sweet Potato
15. Honeydew Melon

- Romaine, Red Leaf, Escarole, or Chicory Lettuce varieties
- Onions (yellow and red)
- Scallions (also known as green onions)
- Green, Red, Yellow, Orange Peppers
- Tomatoes
- Cucumbers
- Cilantro
- Lemons
- Celery
- Potatoes
- Broccoli, Cabbage, Kale, Collard Greens, Turnip Greens, Mustard Greens, or Cauliflower
- Apples, Bananas, Grapes, Citrus Fruits

Meats: (fresh and frozen)
- Wild Caught Fish
- Organic or No Antibiotic/No Hormone Chicken, Lamb, Beef
- Turkey Sausage or Bacon with No Nitrites or No Nitrates

Dairy Section:
- Organic Yogurt or Greek Yogurt
- Organic Butter (NO NO NO Spread, Margarine, Butter infused w/ oils, I Can't Believe It's Not Butter)
- Soft Cheeses

- Organic Milk (If you can't make the run to a local farm for fresh milk, most health food stores carry a local brand. However, in a pinch organic milk is still better than regular milk.)
- Organic Eggs or No Antibiotic/No Hormone Eggs

<u>Bakery:</u>
- Multi-Grain Bread with Unbleached Unbromated Flour (An excellent brand is Wegman's *Food You Feel Good About* MultiGrain Bread), Rye Bread, or Wheat Bread without High Fructose Corn Syrup

We should come to the understanding that we do not have to buy ten apples at once nor a 20-pound sack of potatoes—unless you are feeding a pack with bottomless pits—because fresh food and organic food does not last as long.

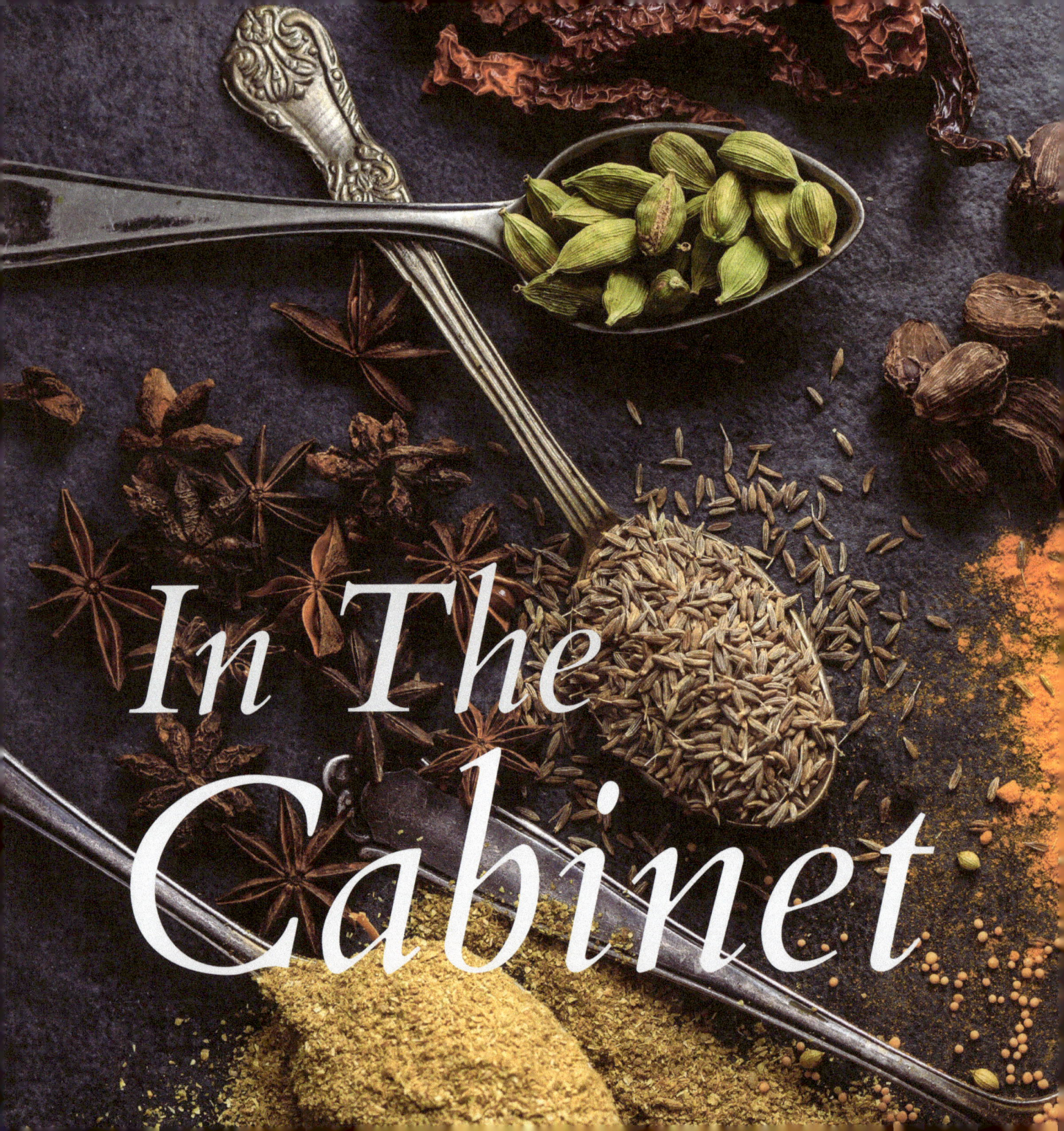

The following is a list of items that should be staples in your Healing and Detox Laboratory—the Kitchen.

DRY SEASONINGS:

Most of these products are organic and really do the job in the flavor enhancing department AND not as much is needed. My favorite brand is Simply Organic followed by Frontier. If you have to go conventional, buy the McCormick brand.

- Cayenne Pepper
- Celery Salt
- Chilli Powder
- Cinnamon
- Cloves (Ground and Whole)
- Cream of Tartar
- Dry Mustard
- Fines Herbs
- Garlic Powder
- Ground Cumin
- Herbs du Provence
- Himalayan Salt
- Morjam (Fresh, Dried)
- Nutmeg
- Old Bay Seasoning
- Onion Powder
- Oregano (Fresh, Dried)
- Paprika (Smoked, Hungarian)

- Parsley (Fresh, Dried)
- Rosemary (Fresh, Dried)
- Saffron
- Sage (Ground, Dried)
- Sea Salt
- Thyme (Ground, Fresh, Dried)
- Vege-Sal (replaces seasoning salt)

LIQUIDS:

- Extra Virgin Olive Oil (First Cold Press)
- Bragg's Liquid Aminos (replaces soy sauce)
- Bragg's Apple Cider Vinegar with the 'Mother'
- White Wine Sherry
- Red Wine Sherry
- Bar-B-Que Sauce
- Louisiana One-Drop-Does-It Hot Sauce
- Newman's Salad Dressings (these contain NO MSG nor High Fructose Corn Syrup)
- Sesame Oil (Light and Dark)

Now that you have decided to change over the pantry to healthy items—especially to items that contain NO MSG—when shopping and reading labels learn to watch for these ingredients listed below which do contain MSG. Many manufacturers know that we know MSG should be avoided so, instead of listing MSG as an ingredient they use these ingredients which contain MSG instead.

Kitchen Warriors 101: Homemade Healthy

The MSG Masquerade:
Foods to Avoid Containing MSG

Anything Enzyme Modified
Anything Protein Fortified
Anything Ultra-Pasteurized
Autolyzed Yeast
Bouillon
Broth
Calcium Calceinate
Carrageenan
Citric Acid
Corn Starch
Enzymes
Gelatin
Glutamate
Glutamate Acid
Hydrolyzed Protein
Malt
Malt Extract

Malt Flavoring
Maltodextrin
Monopotassium Glutamate
Monosodium Glutamate
Natural Beef Flavoring
Natural Chicken Flavoring
Natural Flavorings/Seasonings
Natural Pork Flavoring
Pectin Powdered Milk
Protease
Soy Protein
Soy Protein Isolate
Soy Sauce
Stock
Textured Protein
Yeast Extract
Yeast Food and Nutrient

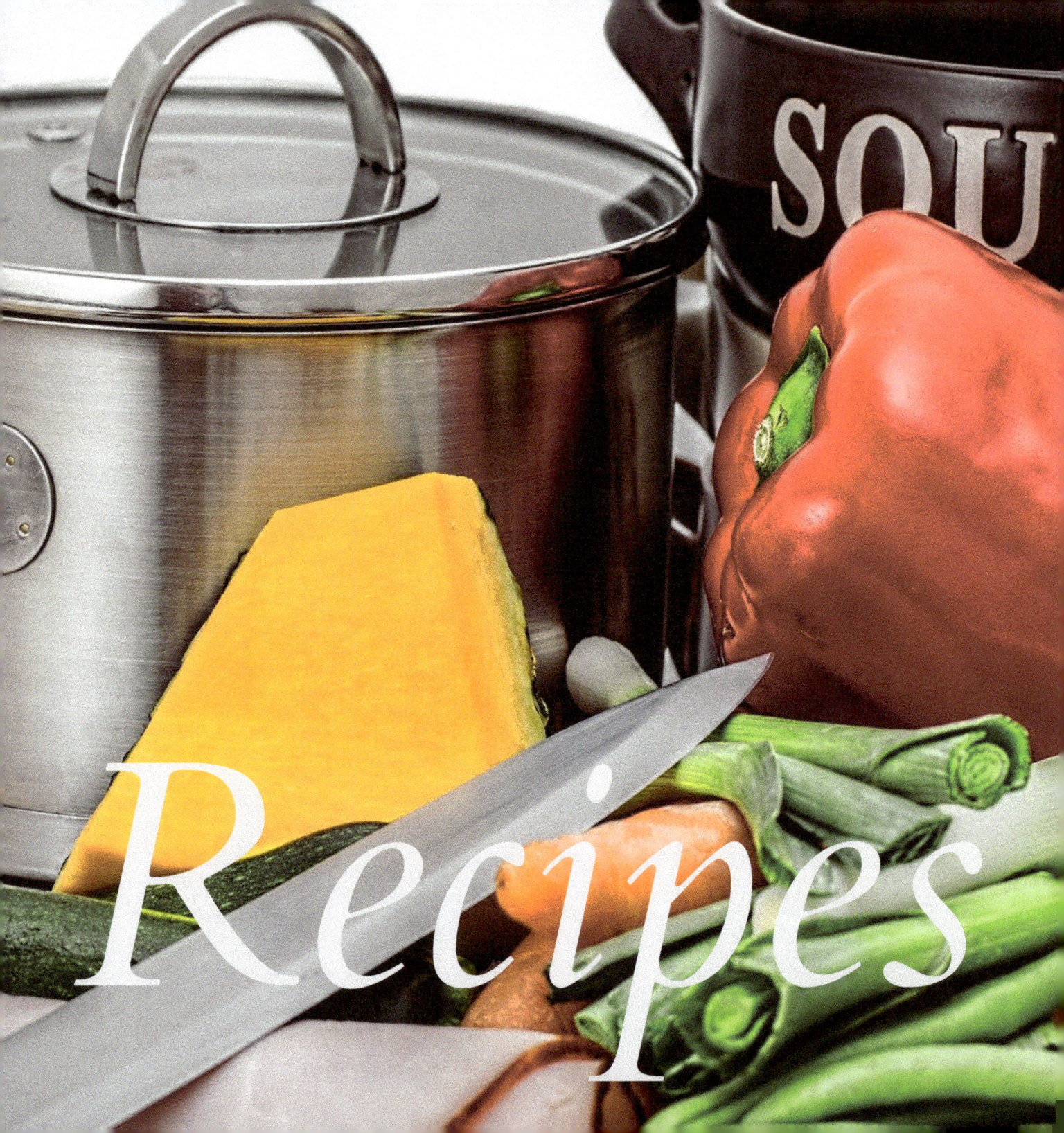

Lord, we thank you for the food we are about to receive for the nourishment of our bodies. Thank you for the hands that have prepared it. Amen

— Traditional prayer

The recipes listed on these pages are enjoyed regularly by my family and friends. I am asked every single day when I teach or give someone an alternate eating plan, "Dr. Brookshire, what do YOU eat?" I have to admit that I absolutely LOVE food, I mean I LOVE food and I did NOT accumulate the "junk in my trunk" from eating just carrots! Fortunately, I like the preparation of food as much as eating. I have discovered that chopping and dicing soothes my soul. Many of my friends insist I must have too much time on my hands to come up with these tasty recipe variations and they have nicknamed me "The Black Martha Stewart".

I have to thank my Daddy Bo for being a willing participant in all of the items I have 'concocted' over the years, for submitting to our every whim of the goodies we have seen on TV, and for eating each bite with joy! Every girl who likes to whip things up in the kitchen needs a willing participant to eat and a willing participant who will do the shopping –no matter the hour—when you say, "If you go to the store, I'll make it."

A lot of these recipes were inspired by dishes I love that were prepared in restaurants and at the hands of family and friends. I am not embarrassed to call the chief from a restaurant kitchen to ask about ingredients, nor am I to ask to swap a recipe with friends. Many of my girlfriends and I have great joy in swapping recipes and showing off our latest cookbooks. We spend many hours copying recipes from the books we share with one another. Here are more than more than 100 of my favorites that I cook over-and-over and have perfected my way.

Please note: I enjoy my food with intense flavors. My family loves to taste their food in the same way. That said, some of the quantities of seasonings may seem a little much. Try just a pinch of something you are not sure about or halving a spice that you may not want to taste as much of in the dish. I have never had any complaints from anyone at my table only, Oh-my-goodness-this-is-sooooooo-good compliments.

My suggestion is that you start fresh, and use organic to get the same results. If you cannot always get organics, Always buy real food—not fake food replacements, i.e. margarine, artificial sweeteners, vegetable oils, spray oils, or items that have ingredients you cannot pronounce.

Real food always garners real results which equals delicious. Use these recipes to put together a daily meal plan to accomplish good health:

5 Fruits
5 Vegetables
2 Proteins
2 Starches

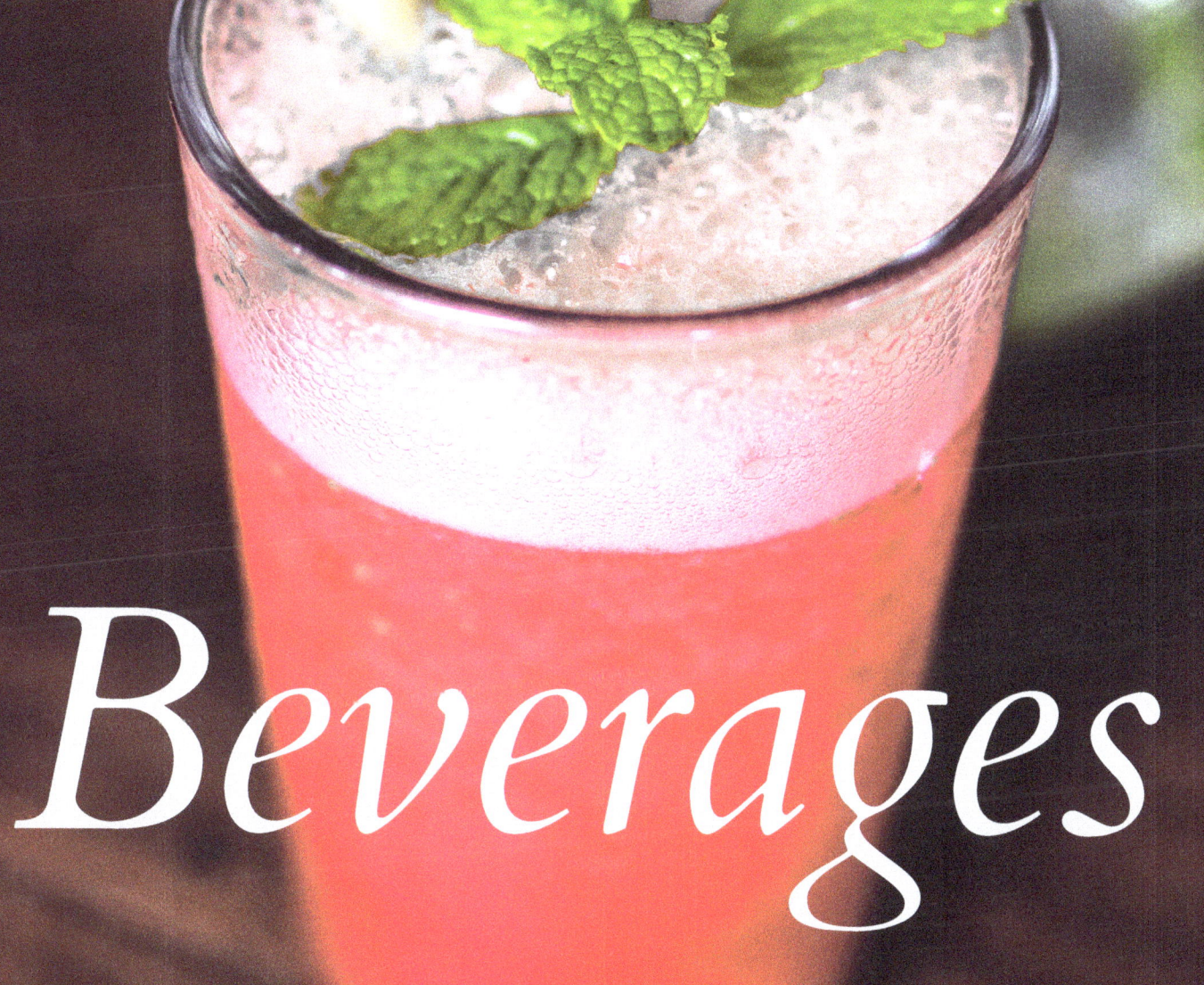

Beverages

Dr. LaJoyce Brookshire

Fruit Water – "The Real Fruit 2 O"

-cut up fresh fruit in dices and layer the bottom of a pitcher about 2 inches
(Watermelon, Peaches, Berries, Mango, Lemons/Oranges are best)
-pour filtered water over the fruit
-refrigerate overnight
-the water will totally take on the flavor of the fruit

Fruit Water Variations:
-cut up both Lemons and Oranges with the rind
-1 Tablespoon of Cloves
or
-Celery chopped
or
-Cucumber chopped
or
-Ginger chopped
These waters are excellent for guests as an alternative beverage.

Nutritional Note:
Celery and Cucumber waters are totally refreshing, hydrating, and detoxifying. Ginger helps to stimulate enzymes in the pancreas and kills harmful bacteria thereby aiding in digestion.

beverages

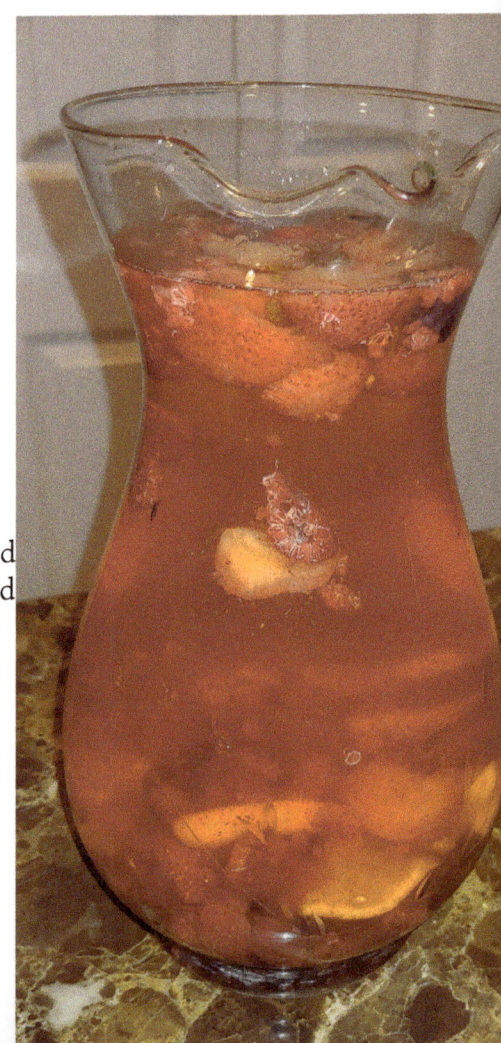

The Green Morning Drink

1 cup Organic Spinach (can also use Cabbage or Kale)
1 rib Organic Celery
3-4 sprigs Cilantro or Parsley (both if need to detoxify)
½ Lemon seeded with the yellow cut-off leaving as much white as possible
1 Tablespoon Green Vibrance Multi-Vitamin/Multi-Mineral Formula
20-24 oz water
Ice (optional)

-chop all items and place in blender
-liquefy until all is smooth
-drink immediately
-can be kept in fridge for up to 24 hours

Tips:
-Pre-package in a freezer Ziploc all items chopped and ready to blend
-Drink before 3pm as this drink gives you energy
-Drink immediately after blending – this is not a sip-like-tea beverage

Nutritional Note:
The Green Morning Drink is a great way to start the day. It detoxifies the body gently and naturally. The combination of Cilantro and Parsley removes heavy metal toxicity. Amazing weight loss benefits have been reported.

-Do NOT get creative by adding fruit other than lemon to this recipe as fruit should not mix with these veggies. Use exactly as here for maximum health benefits.

Fruit Smoothie

Cut-up fruit and freeze in Ziplocs (no need to use ice w/ frozen fruit)
2-3 frozen fruits in blender (i.e. Banana, Strawberries, Pineapple – any combination)
1 container of organic yogurt (optional)
1 Tablespoon Flax Seeds or Chia Seeds (optional)
1 Tablespoon Green Vibrance (a multi-vitamin/multi-mineral supplement)
½ cup organic apple juice
½ cup water

-Blend and enjoy for breakfast or anytime.

Nutritional Note:
Smoothies are a great way to usher in perfect health. Just about any fruit or vegetable can be put into a smoothie to help an ailment or for enjoyment. My favorite blender is the Blend-Tec which can pulverize an avocado seed to dust. If the cost is out of reach, a 14-speed Oster with the glass pitcher is a good place to start, as well as the Ninja, or Magic Bullet.

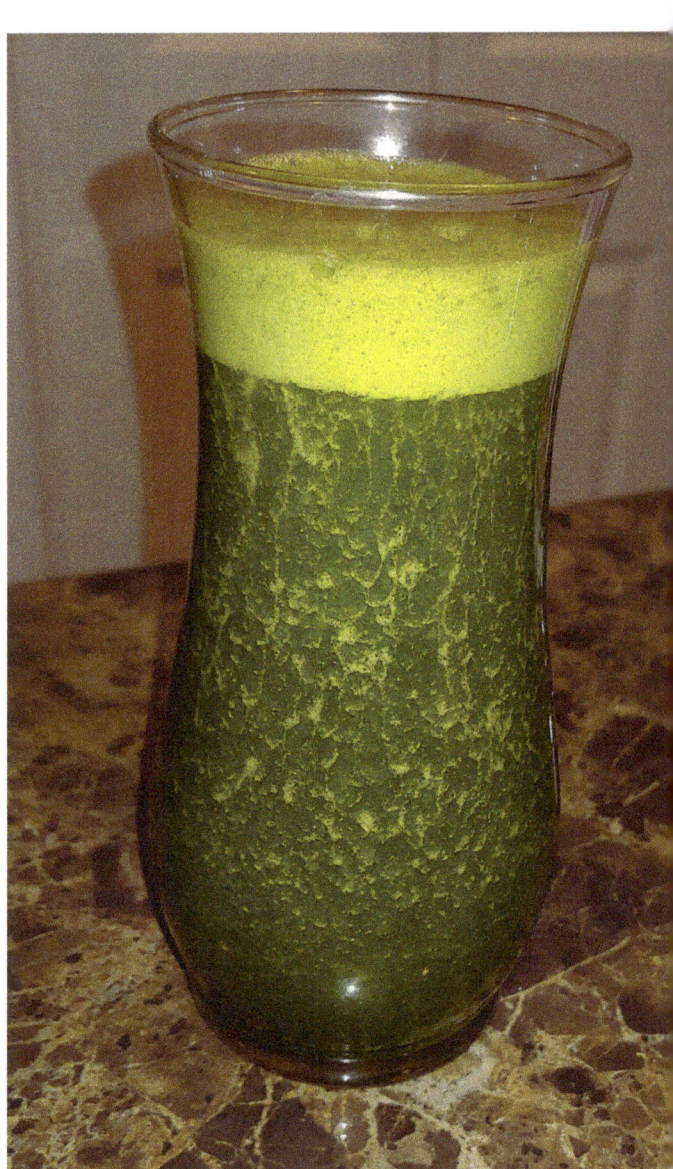

Hot Cocoa

1 ½ cups milk
1 Tablespoon Carob Powder
1 Tablespoon Raw Honey
½ teaspoon Vanilla

-Heat until warm and serve.

Hot Apple Cider

2 cups organic Apple Cider
1 Cinnamon Stick
Pinch of Nutmeg

-Heat until hot and serve in a mug with a pinch of Nutmeg on top and submerge the Cinnamon Stick.

Dr. LaJoyce Brookshire

Eggnog
(non-alcoholic)

12 eggs separated
1 cup sugar
1/8 teaspoon Sea Salt
4 Tablespoons Vanilla Extract
2 Tablespoons Rum Extract
1 Tablespoon Almond Extract
1 quart Heavy Whipping Cream
1 quart Half & Half
2 Tablespoons Nutmeg
4 Tablespoons Cinnamon
A long handled wooden spoon
A slotted spoon

Warning: this recipe GROWS in quantity exponentially so use an 8 quart container from the beginning.

-in a mixing bowl beat egg whites until stiff
-beat in ½ cup sugar
-in the 8 quart container beat yolks with the wooden spoon
-mix in ½ cup sugar and salt until light in color
-combine egg mixtures and mix thoroughly with the wooden spoon
-in mixing bowl beat heavy cream* until thick and creamy

Watch this process closely! Over-whipping of the cream will result in it turning to butter. If this happens, add a couple pinches of Himalayan Salt, mix, place in a container and use it for butter.

-add all of the extracts and Half and Half, blend with wooden spoon
-add cinnamon and nutmeg using the slotted spoon until creamy
-the eggnog will be heavy and tight when it is first made and needs to be shaken and stirred often
-refrigerate for at least one day before drinking to chill
-if eggnog needs to be served before sitting, shake every 10-15 minutes for ingredients to blend into one another. The 8 quart quantity will eventually melt down to about half.
-may add libations to individual cups

Hand-Squeezed Lemonade

I prefer to hand-squeeze because I like the pulp. To avoid pulp, juice the lemons instead.

12 Lemons
Honey to taste
-Garnish with a Fruit Ice Cubes (see recipe)

Variation:
-Blend fresh Ginger Root and add to Lemonade for an extra flavor and health enhancer.

Fruit Ice Cubes
2-3 cups of fruits like Strawberries, Pears, Mangos, Watermelon, Peaches
1 cup water
-blend until smooth in blender
-spoon into ice cube trays
-when frozen, place into Ziploc bags
-add 2-3 fruit ice cubes to a glass and pour Lemonade or Iced Tea on top

Watermelon Lime-Aid Slushy

During watermelon season, I purchase two at a time. One to eat, and one to freeze. There is nothing more refreshing than sweet, sweet watermelon in the winter months. I also only purchase watermelons WITH seeds because I always ask, "How'd they grow that?!" Well… I know the answer but that is another book.

Nutritional Note:
Eat as much watermelon as possible in season as it is the king of all fruit, and the black seeds are a powerful kidney cleanser.

1 whole Watermelon with frozen into cubes
2 limes
2 Tablespoons Organic Cane Sugar or Raw Honey
2 cups water

-cut limes in half and cut-off all of the green leaving the white and put in blender first
-add sugar
-fill a blender almost to the top with frozen watermelon cubes
-pour water on top
-blend until smooth
-serve in frosted glasses garnished with a slice of lime
* Buy watermelons in season

Coco Colada

1 can Coconut Crème
2 cups cubed fresh frozen Pineapple (can add strawberries)
2 cups water

-put all ingredients in blender
-liquefy until smooth
-serve with a wedge of Pineapple or Strawberry

Baby Formula

I fed my baby girl Brooke this formula as a supplement to breast feeding and then gave her this recipe exclusively when she was weaned. This mixture is an immune booster and easily replaces canned baby formulas. This may seem like a bit of a project for the first few attempts, but trust me it gets easier and your baby will love the taste!

1 cup Organic hulled barley or organic barley
4 quarts of Filtered water from a Brita or Pur Water Filter System
Myenberg Powdered Goat Milk

Organic brown rice syrup
Cheese cloth
New Rubbermaid 4 quart pitcher
New wooden spoon
New stainless strainer
New designated soup pot - either stainless steel or glass

-double the cheese cloth into a square
-place 1 cup of barley in the center of the cloth
-loosely tie the ends together so that no barley can fall out
(the barley will swell and that's why the cloth should be loose)
-fill soup pot with 4-5 quarts of filtered water
*do NOT use bottled water.
-drop the cloth with barley into the filled pot
-cook covered on low heat about 1 hour until the water turns a brownish pink
-take off of stove and allow water to cool down to warm in the pot
-strain the water into the Rubbermaid pitcher
-if you have 3 or 4 quarts of water measure the appropriate amount of goat milk for that quantity and add it to the liquid - stir until dissolved
-add just enough brown rice syrup to notice there is a HINT of sweet
-fill a bottle or two to have handy and refrigerate the rest in the pitcher
-using the wooden spoon, stir the contents in the pitcher before pouring into a bottle
-warm the bottle using a bottle warmer or by placing bottle in a bowl with hot water
-formula stays fresh for no more than 3 days.

beverages

NEVER USE THE MICROWAVE TO HEAT THE FORMULA for this destroys the nutritional content of the formula and ANY other food for that matter!

Nutritional Note:

-the barley is loaded with iron and other minerals necessary for baby's growth
-the filtered water is from a flowing source and not stagnant in plastic bottles that have been sitting on store shelves
-this is a great supplement to breast feeding and can be given to baby up until 2-years-old.
-the barley in the cheese cloth can be eaten by you or once baby begins to eat food like oatmeal only when baby can sit-up alone. Sweeten it with brown sugar, or the rice syrup and add fresh fruit. Really yummy.

Anti-Plague Formula

This is a tonic that will heal any icky thing that may find its way in to your body. It is awesome for keeping the immune system healthy and strong. My family has been taking the Anti-Plague Formula for many years and it has done the job in times of illness and kept us well during Cold & Flu season. I was pleased to discover that this recipe is an ages old ancient remedy which continues to prove that we have everything we need right in God's garden to be our pharmacy. I learned how to make this tonic from one of the greatest teachers I have ever known, Dr. Michael Vincent. Until now, I have only made this product available in my Wellness Centers or at speaking engagements. During the times we live in today, I find it imperative to share this perfected recipe publicly with you.

Make in a 1 gallon GLASS Jug (THIS MIXTURE WILL MELT PLASTIC!)
24 Habanero Peppers
2 White Onions
1 big Horse Radish or 2 medium
2 Ginger Roots
12-18 Garlic bulbs (50-60 cloves total)
1 gallon Bragg's Raw Apple Cider Vinegar "with the Mother"
(buy 4 - 32oz bottles and save the bottles for storage)

USING LATEX GLOVES:
-cut all ingredients one at a time into small pieces using either a food processor or knife
-shove the pieces into the glass jug
(I like to use a large funnel that I have chopped off the tip for easy shoving)
-when everything is cut-up and put into the jug, notice that the jug will be almost filled with the goodies
-add the Apple Cider Vinegar until the jug is just about filled. Leave a bit of room for the mixture to be able to move around.
-will only be able to use about 2 ½ bottles of the Apple Cider Vinegar, save the remaining vinegar
-shake mixture EVERYDAY for 3 weeks and store in a cool dark place.
After 3 Weeks:
- strain the liquid with a new strainer into a large pot
-empty out the sediment into a large glass bowl or pot to reserve it
-juice the sediment 2x and pour into the large pot with the other liquid – this process should yield another 2 cups or more of liquid
 pour the finished Anti-Plague product back into the Vinegar bottles for easy usage and storage
-top off the bottles with vinegar

-dilute the 32oz bottles even further with 1-32oz bottle of Vinegar
-make a label with the date made or follow the expiration date on the Vinegar bottle– the longer Anti-Plague sits, the more potent it becomes
-when there are 2 diluted bottles left, start the process all over again

(I save some of the sediment to use in soups or to sautee in to recipes. Freeze the sediment in 2 tablespoon quantities in BPA-Free plastic bags or freeze it in ice trays)
-Feel Free to sell 1 – 32oz bottle for at least $100

-Store in a cool dark place in Glass ONLY - -This mixture will MELT PLASTIC!!!
-Do not refrigerate to allow moisture into the mixture!!
-This mixture will MELT PLASTIC!!!
-ALWAYS take with food
-take 1 tablespoon per day for prevention – 1 teaspoon for children
-take 1 shot glass per day or more if infected with ANY virus until symptoms subside
-take 1 shot glass when a cold is coming or with a fever
-helps to combat: any infections, any Virus, and to keep immune system strong
-if infected, take before going to bed and NEVER go to bed KNOWING you do not feel well

Nutritional Note:
These items combined have anti-inflammatory, anti-fungal, anti-bacterial, anti-parasitic, and disinfectant power. If there is a little bugger trying to take hold of you, Anti-Plague Formula will handle it! This tonic is HOT with flavor yet it will not damage the digestive tract, stomach or esophageal lining. In fact, after the initial 'burn', chase it with water and food then experience soothing relief due to the Apple Cider Vinegar balancing the stomach's pH level by neutralizing acid in the stomach. To stay on the side of Prevention, take 1 Tablespoon daily and experience Perfect Health.

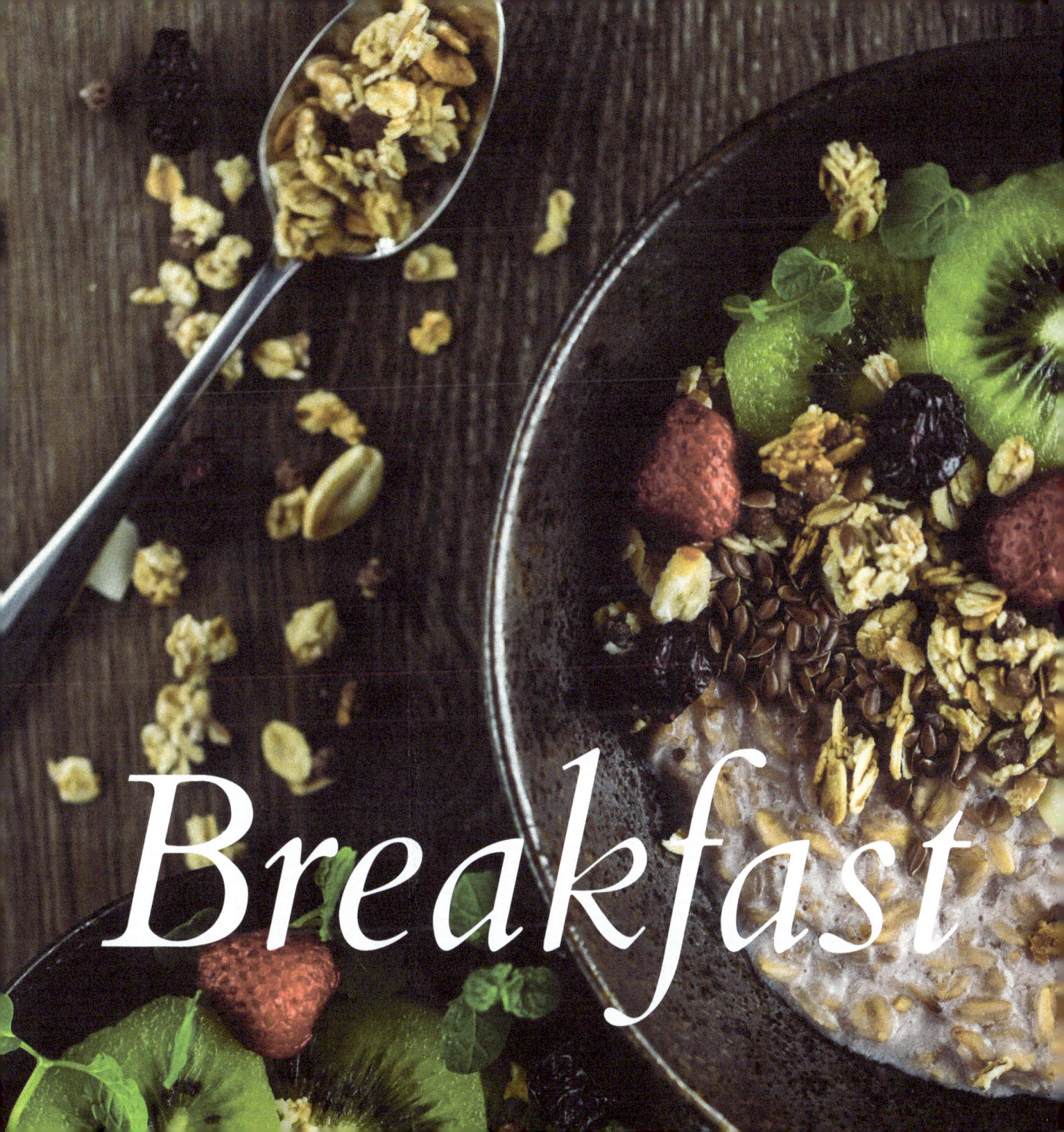

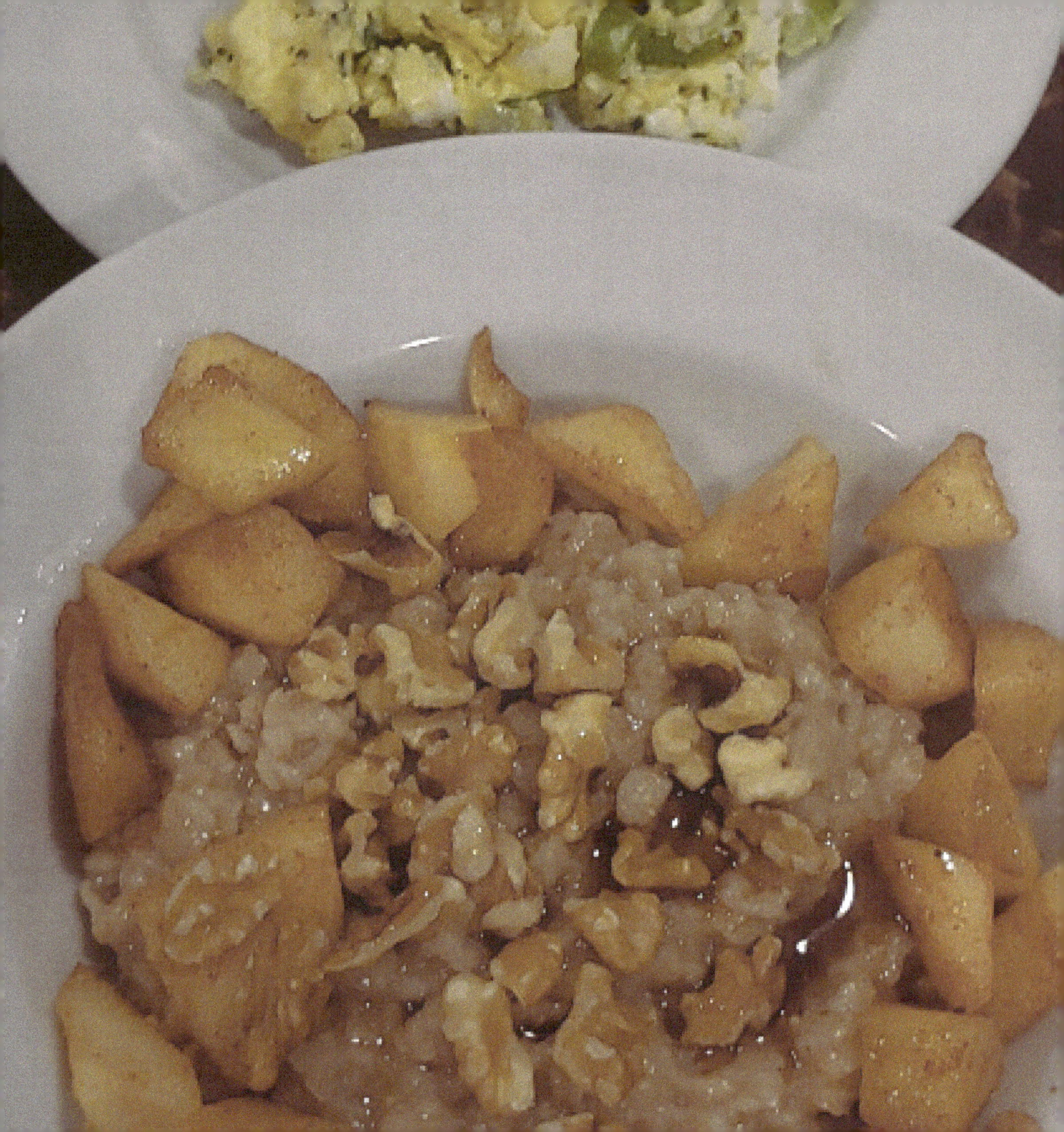

Oatmeal

1 cup organic Oatmeal
1 cup organic Raw Milk
1 cup water (can vary depending on desired soupiness)
2 teaspoons Vanilla Extract
1 teaspoon raw Honey or organic Maple Syrup to taste
1 apple peeled, cored, chopped
2 pats butter

-bring milk, water, vanilla to a boil
-add oatmeal and cook 6-10 minutes
-while oatmeal cooks, prepare apple. In a sauté pan melt 1 pat of butter with vanilla extract
-when bubbling occurs add apples and toss to coat thoroughly
-stir in a pat of butter to the cooked oatmeal
-place apples in a bowl, pour oatmeal on top
-add maple syrup or honey
-can garnish with raisins, cranberries, or walnuts

Grits

3 cups water
½ teaspoon Vege-Sal
5 Tablespoons Bob's Red Mill Organic Yellow Grits
(once you taste organic yellow grits, you will never go back to white)

- bring Vege-Sal water to a boil
- spoon in grits and stir
- lower heat to cook until water boils out
- stir frequently and the grits will bulk-up
- can add more water to reach desired consistency
- serve with a pat of butter on top and a sprinkle of Cayenne Pepper*

Nutritional Note:
Use Cayenne Pepper instead of Black Pepper as it scratches the Liver.

Variations:
Can add sautéed Onions, Mushrooms, assorted Peppers, Celery to put atop the Grits.

Or…Can sautee Shrimp, Scallops or Turkey Keilbasa on them as well… Oh, My Goodness…It is so good!

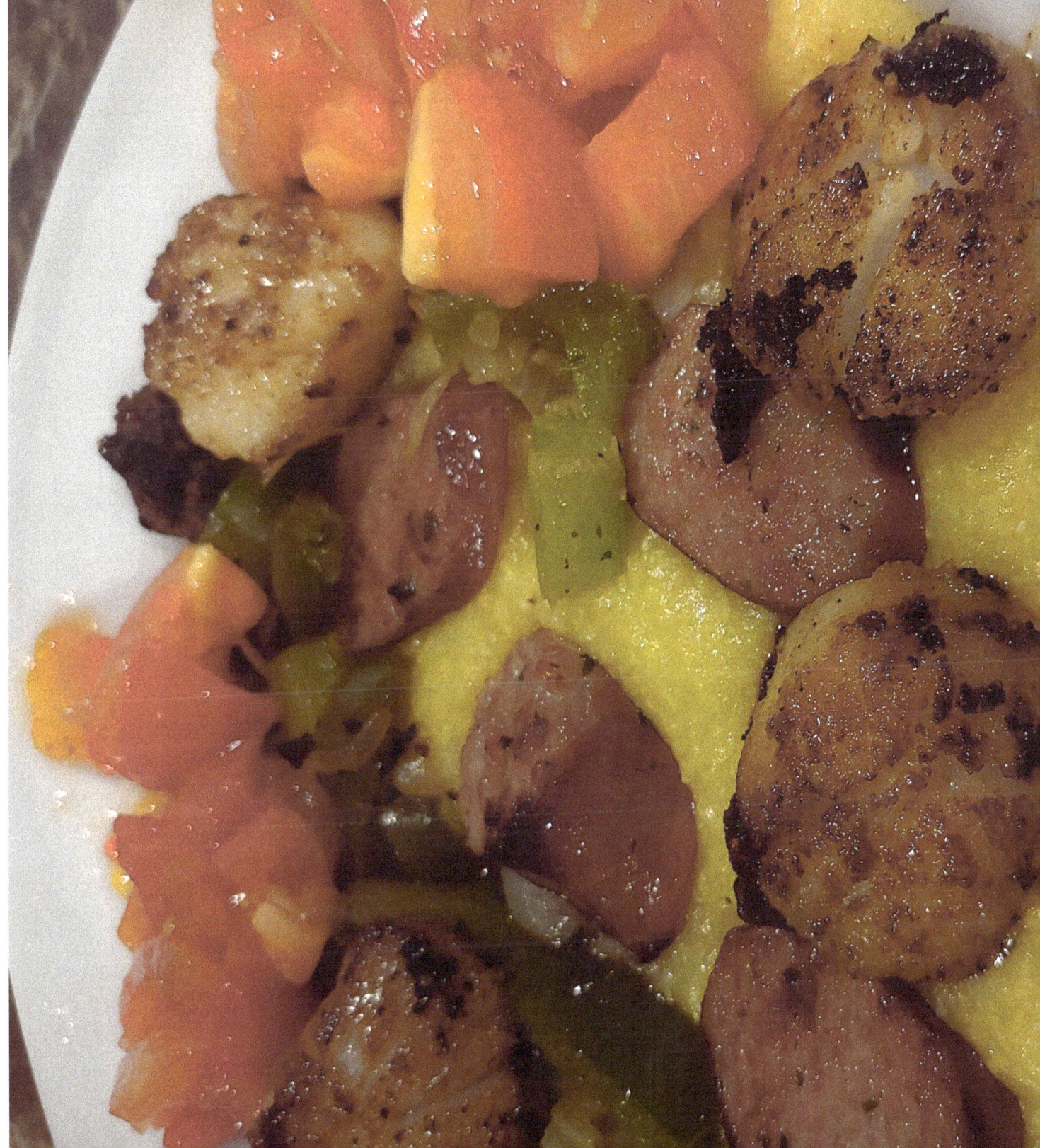

Dr. LaJoyce Brookshire

Egg Omelet

2 Eggs
½ cup scallions or yellow onions
½ cup chopped tomatoes
Sprinkles of Goat Cheese
Pinches of Parsley
Pinch of Vege-Sal
Pinch of Cayenne
Extra-Virgin Olive Oil

-heat oil in the skillet
-meanwhile chop tomatoes and scallions or onions, put in pan and sauté
-beat eggs and pour evenly on top of vegetables
-sprinkle Vege-Sal, cheese, parsley on top
-cook slowly to allow cheese to melt
-fold egg in half when the top is no longer runny
-slide onto plate and enjoy with slices of avocado and tomato

Smothered Potatoes and Onions

4-5 potatoes
Yellow onions
1 teaspoon Vege-Sal or to taste
1 Tablespoon Garlic Powder
1 teaspoon Onion Powder
1 handful Parsley
Extra Virgin Olive oil to coat the skillet + ¼ cup water

-make ¼ inch potato slices – keep skin on!
-put in olive oil over medium heat with all of the seasonings and toss to coat with the oil
-slice the onions thinly using enough to cover all of the potatoes
-the potatoes will begin to get soft and as they do turn them over to marry with the onions
-cook until fork tender and begin to turn slightly brown

Pan Fried Toast

This family tradition is a nod to my Uncle Major who whips-up all sort of delicacies that are perfected by him alone. In my effort to enjoy this toast in a healthy way, this is my yummy modification.

1 Tablespoon Coconut Oil
2 slices Multi-Grain or Ezekiel Bread

-heat cast iron pan
-smear Coconut Oil on both sides of the bread
-place bread on hot pan and toast both sides

Nutritional Note:
Coconut Oil is a delicious and nutritious alternative to butter. It is a good fat which has many health benefits including restoring memory.

Ezekiel Bread is a Biblical bread based on the scripture from Ezekiel 4:9 which states…
Take thou also unto thee wheat, and barley, and beans, and lentils, and millet, and fitches, and put them in one vessel, and make thee bread thereof…

This is a sprouted grain bread and is best kept in the freezer until ready for use as it has no artificial ingredients and spoils quickly. The texture is coarse and holds up well for hearty sandwiches. The fiber quotient for two slices is 6g which is a great contributor for the daily recommended dosage.

Cranberry Banana Bran Muffins
(On the cover)

2-3 Bananas ripened and mashed
1 cup Bob's Red Mill Wheat Bran
1 ½ cups Bob's Red Mill Whole Wheat Flour (or any other brand)
1 teaspoon Aluminum Free Baking Powder
1 teaspoon Baking Soda
1 cup Organic Coconut Creamer or Coconut Milk or Whole Organic Milk
¾ cup Organic Maple Syrup
¼ cup chopped Nuts (optional)
4 Tablespoons Extra Virgin Olive Oil or Coconut Oil
2 Eggs beaten
1 cup Cranberries thawed

-preheat oven to 400
-blend Bananas until smooth then add Maple Syrup
-mix-in Bran, Flour, Baking Soda, Baking Powder, Oil, Egg, Milk
-fold in Cranberries
-do not over mix
-scoop into greased Muffin tin or paper
-bake for 20 minutes

<u>Nutritional Note:</u>
This yummy treat is a delicious way to increase fiber without noticing. Bake once a week to keep handy as a snack alternative. A great breakfast when paired with Organic Yogurt or a Smoothie.

Turkey Bacon

Applegate Farms has a dynamite Turkey Bacon product that contains No Nitrates, No Nitrites, No Antibiotics and No Hormones. Pork Bacon is the hardest food to give up for the wellness model and many have expressed their disdain for Turkey Bacon. Even if you cannot try the Applegate product, start with Butterball or Oscar Meyer Turkey Bacon.

The trick to enjoying this item is knowing *how* to cook it. Here are some variations:

Pan-Crispy Turkey Bacon
Extra Virgin Olive Oil or Coconut Oil
Turkey Bacon

-heat up oil in skillet on medium heat
-when oil gets hot, add turkey bacon
(Cooking tip is the oil because the turkey bacon does not make oil)
-pan fry until both sides are golden brown and crispy

Oven-Fried Turkey Bacon
Extra Virgin Olive Oil or Coconut Oil
Turkey Bacon

-grease a cookie sheet, lay turkey bacon flat
-using fingers, grease the top of each bacon strip
-cook on high heat 450-550 degrees
-check frequently to avoid burning

Sweet Baked Turkey Bacon
-grease cookie sheet well with Olive Oil or Coconut Oil
-lightly spoon maple syrup, pineapple preserves, or orange marmalade onto bacon and bake DELICIOUS!!

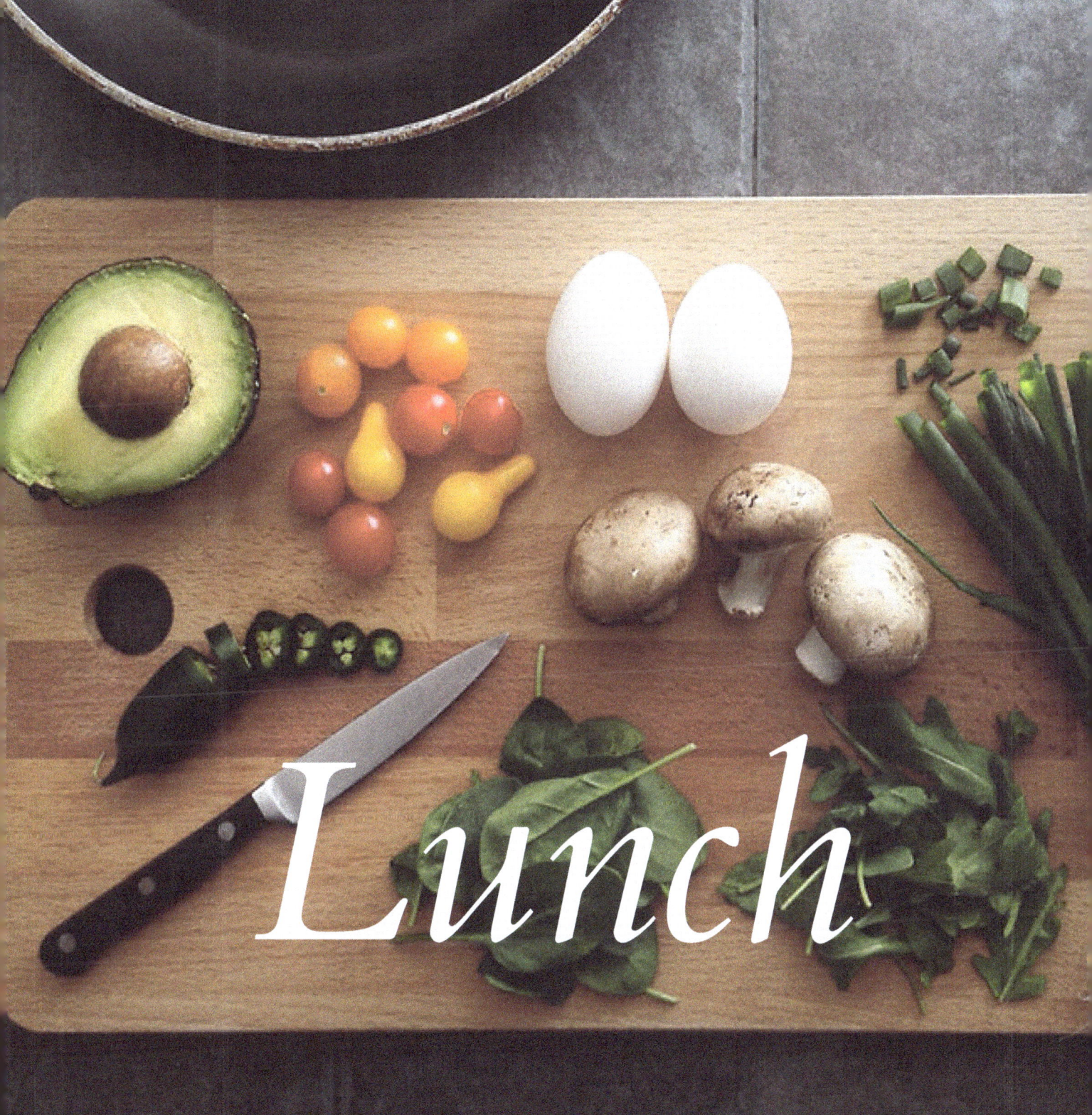

Egg Salad Sandwich

2 hard boiled eggs
2 Tablespoons Miracle Whip
Pinch Vege-Sal
Pinch Parsley
Multi-Grain Bread or bed of salad greens

-chop boiled eggs in a bowl and add Miracle Whip
(yes, Miracle Whip is one of the non-organic products I REFUSE to let go!)
-pinch in Vege-Sal and parsley until reach desired taste
-excellent on a bed of salad greens or as a sandwich with lettuce, tomato, red onion

Nutritional Note:
A good substitute for Miracle Whip is Nayonaise. It is delicious! I think Miracle Whip is my one culinary guilty pleasure. However, Nayonaise is an excellent alternative.

Kitchen Warriors 101: Homemade Healthy

Turkey or Chicken Sandwich

1 Chicken or 1 whole Turkey Breast
Season well – Thyme, Sage, Garlic Powder, Onion Powder, Vege-Sal

-roast turkey or chicken as desired
-slice up the entire bird and keep some in fridge and freezer

Nutritional Note:
Due to the antibiotic content in conventional chicken and turkey, I purchase the entire organic chicken or turkey breast and roast them myself for sandwiches and salad.

Turkey or Chicken Salad

-chop Chicken or Turkey remaining on carcass from carving for sandwiches
-add Miracle Whip, onions, celery, apples
-eat over salad greens

Tuna Salad

High quality canned Tuna
1 Egg
Miracle Whip (quantity as desired)
Onions and Celery
-drain water out of Tuna can
-add chopped egg, onions, celery, Miracle Whip

Nutritional Note:
Be sure to purchase a canned tuna that is wild-caught.

Turkey Patti Melt

1 cooked Turkey Burger
Cheddar, Farmer's, Jarlesberg, or Swiss Cheese
Grilled Onions
Multi-Grain or Ezekiel Bread
Butter

-grill sliced onions in olive oil and put to the side
-make exactly like the grilled cheese above but put cooked burger on top of cheese and add grilled onions on burger

Kitchen Warriors 101: Homemade Healthy

Grilled Cheese with Tomatoes

Cheddar, Farmer's, Jarlesberg, Gouda, or Swiss Cheese
Tomatoes
Multi-Grain or Ezekiel Bread
Butter
Pinch of Basil

-butter one side of 2 pieces of bread
-put butter side down on a hot griddle
-layer cheese onto the top of bread several slices of tomatoes on top with a sprinkle of basil and top off with more cheese
-put the other side of the bread on top of the cheese butter side up and flip when bottom side is brown

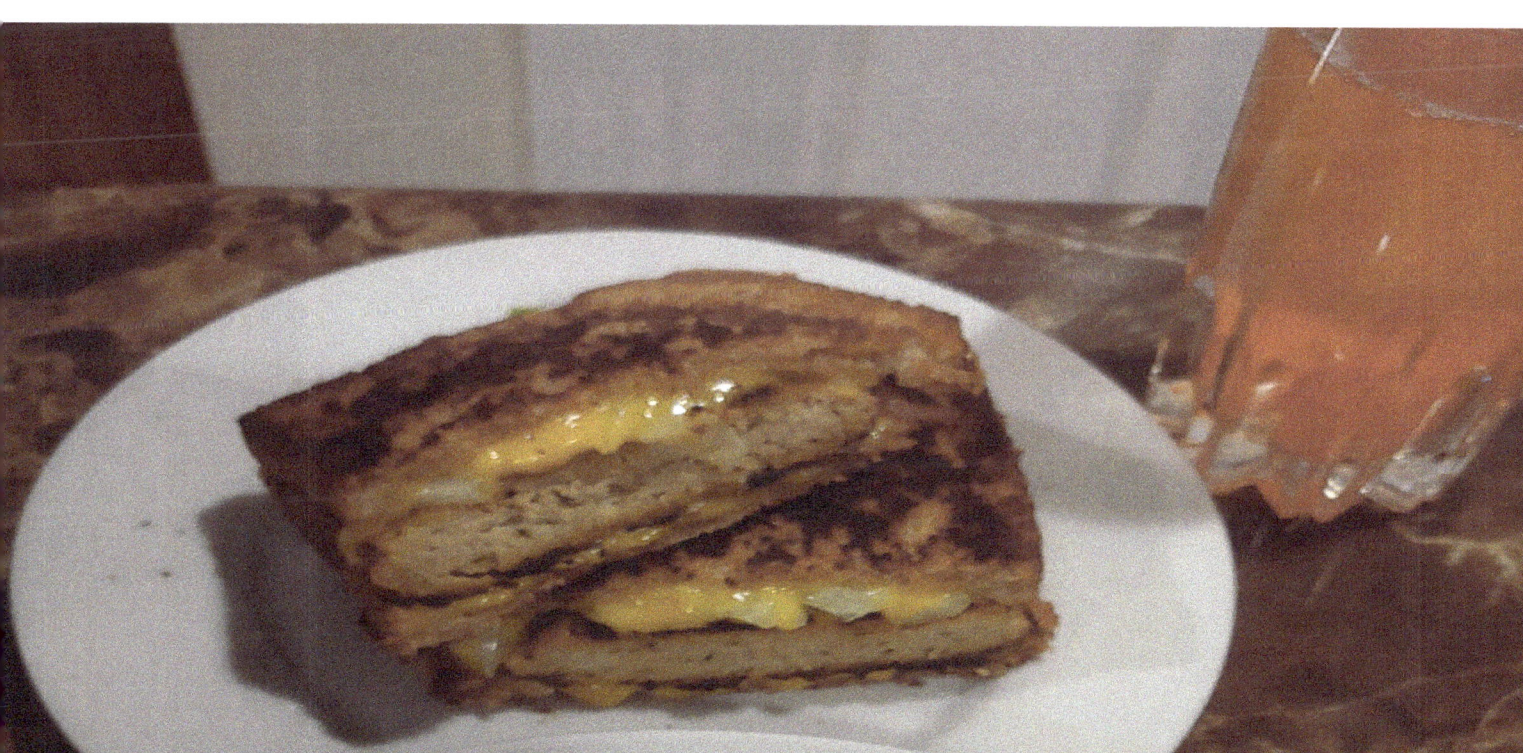

Dr. LaJoyce Brookshire

Rice Noodles with a "Twist"

These packaged noodles are better than the Oodles of Noodles varieties as they contain no MSG.

1 package Rice Noodles
2 Tablespoons Organic Chicken or Lobster Better Than Bouillon
½ each Red, Green, Yellow, Orange Peppers, and Onions
Cooked Chicken, Shrimp, Crab, Scallops (optional)

-boil noodles according to directions
-when reached desired tenderness add Bouillon
-add cooked meat
-add the veggies at the last moment for more than just a noodle meal

Fried Rice

2 cups cooked Brown Basmati Rice, Light Brown Basmati Rice, or Basmati Rice
1 clove Garlic
1 teaspoon shredded Ginger Root (optional)
½ Onion or Scallion (or both)
½ shredded Carrot
½ cup Broccoli
½ cup either Cabbage, Spinach, Kale, Collards, Bok Choy
Handful Ma-Hung Bean Sprouts
¼ cup Bragg's Liquid Aminos
Extra-Virgin Olive Oil
2 Eggs
Parsley

-sauté all veggies in Olive Oil, except Bean Sprouts
-add Rice blending well
-making a hole in the center of the pan, crack 1 Egg in the center and fry on both sides well then blend the rice mix with the egg
-toss in Bean Sprouts
-Liberally adding Parsley
-pour Bragg's Liquid Aminos on top of rice mix well and scoop into bowl
-fry 1 Egg and place on top of rice

Dr. LaJoyce Brookshire

Soft Shell Crab

2 Soft Shell Crabs
1 Egg beaten
2 Tablespoons water
1 cup Yellow Corn Meal
1 teaspoon Vege-Sal or Old Bay
1 teaspoon Garlic Powder
A dash of Cayenne Pepper
Extra Virgin Olive Oil
Cast Iron Skillet

-wash and dry the Crabs
-in a bowl mix Corn Meal, Vege-Sal or Old Bay, Garlic Powder, and Cayenne Pepper
-heat oil in skillet
-beat Egg and water in a bowl large enough for the Crab
-coat crab in the egg mixture
-dunk in Corn Meal completely covering the Crab
-place into hot skillet – do not move crab around
-Crab will begin to crisp-up around edges indicating it is time to flip
-cook until golden brown
-place onto paper towels to drain
-serve on top of a bed of greens with Blue Cheese Cole Slaw (see recipe)
-or-
-serve on a toasted buttered Onion Roll with Blue Cheese Cole Slaw... YUMMY!!!

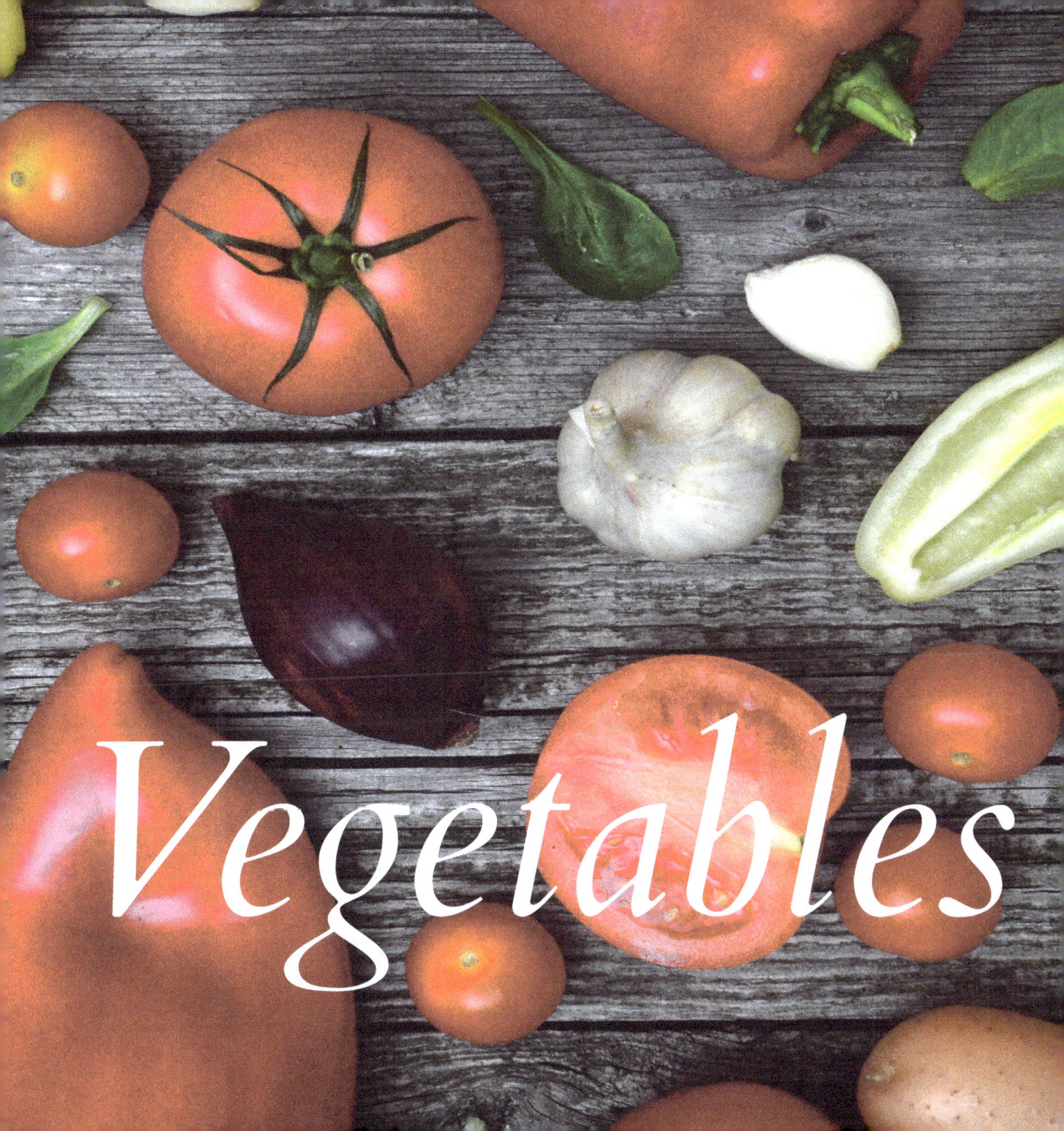

My daughter Brooke has had a love of veggies since she was little. When she was able to get to the stove she wanted to make the Broccoli Rabe so I let her. She makes it so well that mine no longer compares to hers! It has been a delight to enjoy her cooking since she was twelve years old. Brooke not only takes over the cooking of the Rabe, but also Kale, and Spinach.

Nutritional Note:

Not only are various types of greens delicious, they pack a punch in the fiber and chlorophyll departments. While many complain that Broccoli Rabe and Kale are too bitter, these bitter vegetables are the very ones needed to cleanse the blood because they are Astringents. And contains Fiber, Protein, Vitamin C, Vitamin K, and Potassium to name a few.

Broccoli Rabe

1 bunch Broccoli Rabe
Loads of fresh Garlic
¼ cup Extra Virgin Olive Oil
¼ teaspoon Vege-Sal

-sauté garlic in Olive Oil and Vege-Sal until toasted – do not burn Garlic
-clean and chop Broccoli Rabe
-add all of the Rabe to the hot Oil
-will wilt immediately, toss continually to coat

Fresh Spinach

1 container or bunch of fresh Organic Spinach
1-2 chopped Tomatoes

-make exactly like the Broccoli Rabe
-add chopped Tomatoes when cooked

Kale

1 bunch of Kale
½ teaspoon Onion Powder

-make exactly like the Broccoli Rabe
-add Onion Powder

Succotash

2 ears of sweet corn
10 oz fresh Baby Lima Beans (can use frozen)
1 cup fresh chopped Okra
1 ½ cup Milk
Pinch of sweet Basil
Chopped tomatoes (optional)

-cut corn away from cob and boil slowly with Lima Beans in milk
-when corn and beans become tender add okra
-stir in basil and tomatoes when okra is tender

Zucchini and Squash a la "Ma Kitty"

In 2007, I spoke at a church in New Jersey and this dish was on the dinner table untouched. One look and I knew others had NO idea of its deliciousness. I asked the host, "Who made the squash?" She pointed in the kitchen to Ma Kitty. I got the recipe and now I thank her every time I make it.

2 Green Zucchini
2 Yellow Squash
1 Onion
½ Red, Yellow, Green, Orange, Pepper
½ cup water
1 teaspoon Vege-Sal
1 teaspoon Parsley
Pinch of Basil
Extra Virgin Olive Oil

-place Oil, Parsley, Vege-Sal, water in skillet with Zucchini and Squash
-cover and cook until pan begins to steam
-add peppers and Onions on top with another pinch of Vege-Sal and Basil
-cover and cook to just fork tender
-toss to coat blend all items well

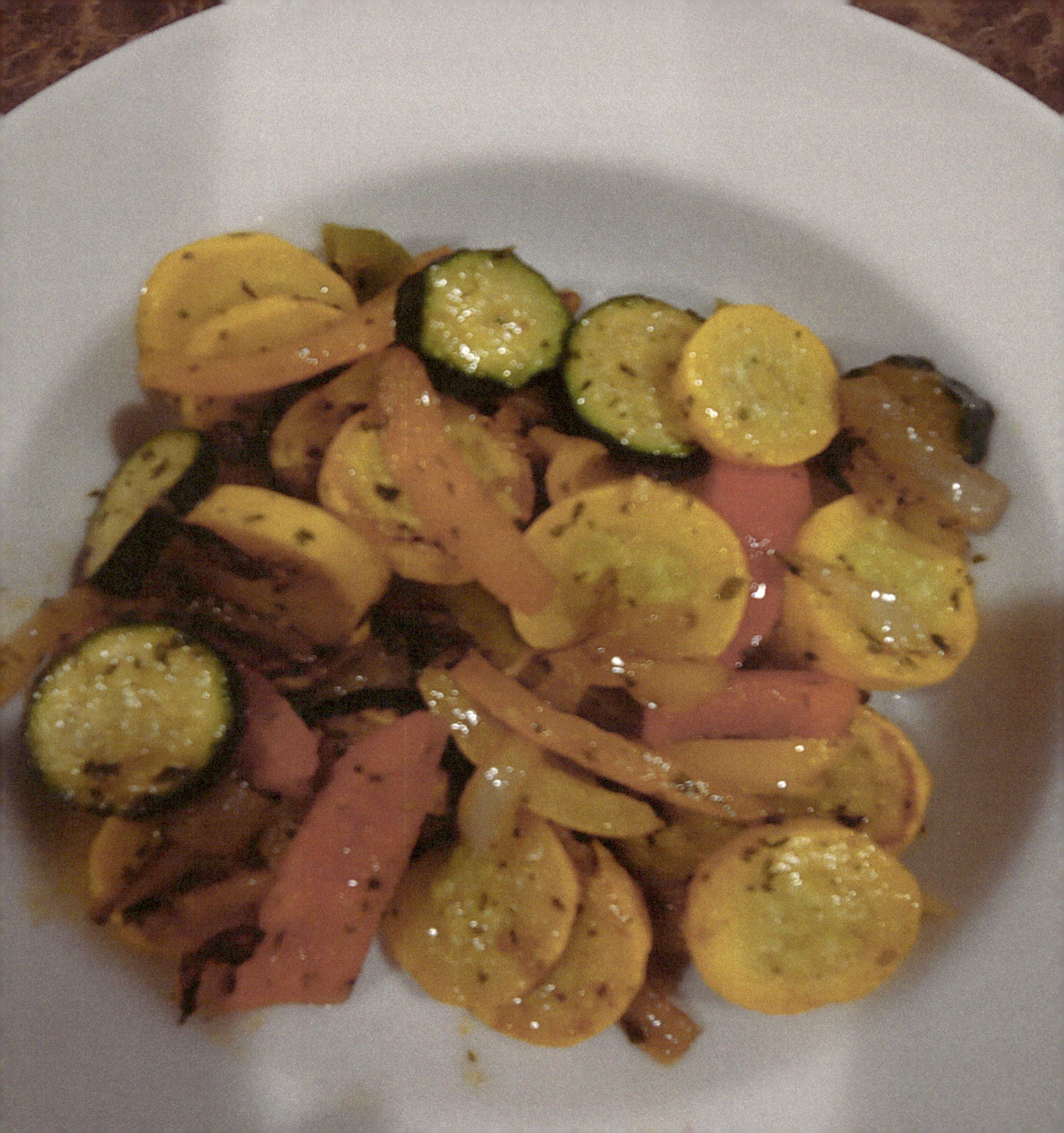

Acorn Squash

2 Acorn Squash
Butter

-preheat oven to 350
-wash Squash well
-grease Squash with Extra Virgin Olive Oil
-place on cookie sheet covered by foil
-when just tender remove from oven and let cool
-cut in half and place face down onto cookie sheet
-once insides are tender scoop out and mash with butter
Or…stuff with sautéed Cauliflower Rice or Wild Rice and Veggies

Butternut Squash

2 Butternut Squash
Cinnamon
Nutmeg
Butter

-cook exactly like the Acorn Squash
-scoop out and mix with Cinnamon, Nutmeg, and Butter to taste

Okra

1 pound Fresh Okra
1 Yellow Onion
1 Tablespoon fresh chopped Garlic
Extra Virgin Olive Oil
¼ teaspoon Basil
¼ teaspoon Thyme
¼ teaspoon Herbs du Provence
1 teaspoon Parsley
¼ teaspoon Vege-Sal

- clean Okra with a damp paper towel by wiping each pod on all sides
- allow to dry lying on a paper toweled cookie sheet not over-lapping this process prevents the slime
- coat bottom of skillet with olive oil layering first garlic, onions, then okra
- sprinkle all seasonings on top
- cook on low heat until Okra is tender but not mushy
- serve on top of Basmati or Brown Rice

Nutritional Note:
The slimy-ness that most folk dislike about Okra is Slippery Elm. Its classification is a Demulcent which soothes the digestive tract. It is wonderful for the body and a delicious hearty vegetable. When anyone yucks the yummy-ness of Okra …I place this dish in front of them.

String Beans and Tomatoes

1 pound String Beans
1 cup cherry tomatoes
Extra Virgin Olive Oil
¼ teaspoon Basil
¼ teaspoon Thyme
¼ teaspoon Rosemary
1 teaspoon Parsley
1 Lemon

-in a steamer steam String Beans until just done to retain a bit of the snap
-in skillet coat with olive oil and all seasonings including the fresh juice of 1 Lemon
-allow herb oil mix to get sizzling hot
-meanwhile, half the Cherry Tomatoes
-remove String Beans from steamer and toss in the sizzling skillet to coat thoroughly
-remove in less than 2 minutes to a serving dish and throw the cold tomatoes on top

String Beans and Boiled Red Potatoes

1 pound String Beans
5 Red Potatoes
1 boiling pot half filled with water (like a soup pot)
2 Tablespoons Better Than Bouillon Organic Chicken Flavored Paste
2 ribs chopped Celery
½ teaspoon Vege-Sal
¼ teaspoon Basil
¼ teaspoon Thyme
¼ teaspoon Rosemary
1 teaspoon Parsley
2 Bay Leaves
Few shakes of Hot Sauce

-bring water and all seasonings to a rolling boil on high heat
-taste the water to determine satisfaction before adding beans
-snap off the tips of Green Beans and add to the rolling boil
-cover and lower heat to medium and cook until just done
-add peeled and halved potatoes to the pot and submerge under water
-turn off the pot and leave on the stove
This is a meal all by itself. Serve with hot cornbread (see recipe under sides).

Meatless "Mean" Collard Greens

2-3 bunches Collard Greens
2 cubed Turnips or ½ chopped Rutabaga
1-2 Tablespoons Garlic Powder
1-2 Tablespoons Onion Powder
1 chopped White or Yellow Onion
2 fresh chopped cloves of garlic
1 Tablespoon Vege-Sal
¼ cup Hot Sauce
2 Tablespoons Extra-Virgin Olive Oil
Pinch of Sugar
Pinch of Nutmeg
1 full soup pot of water

-put cubed Turnips or Rutabaga in water and bring to a rolling boil
(This process is called creating "Pot Liquor".)
-scoop out Turnips or Rutabaga and add all of the seasonings except oil and sugar
-bring water to a rolling boil
-clean greens one leaf at a time front and back a couple of times to ensure all grit and bugs are gone
-layer Greens one over the other -largest to smallest- on a cutting board
-roll greens tightly making 1 inch slices

-place shreds into a bowl until filled and put in boiling water one bowl at a time
-cook on high heat with top off
-when placing each bowl of shredded Greens in the boiling water submerge the new batch
-when reached desired tenderness turn off the stove and add Olive Oil, sugar, and nutmeg
-stir in and leave on stove overnight, and refrigerate in the morning
-Serve with hot Cornbread (see Sides)

Turnip and Mustard Greens Mixed

-Make exactly like Collard Greens above
-Mustard Greens are more labor intensive to clean due to their curliness
-this mix cooks quickly – do NOT overcook!

Cabbage

1 head of Cabbage
1 chopped Onion
1 cup Water
2 Tablespoons Better Than Bouillon Organic Chicken Bouillon Paste
2 teaspoons butter
2 Tablespoons Parsley
¼ teaspoon Basil
Pinch of Organic Cane Sugar

-chop Cabbage into 1 inch shreds
-in a soup pot heat water, Chicken Bouillon, and Onion
-when bouillon melts into water add entire Cabbage
-put chopped Onion on top and sprinkle Basil
-Cabbage will make its own water so cover the pot and cook on medium heat
-toss the Cabbage occasionally until desired tenderness is reached
-when it is done, add Butter and Sugar

Nutritional Note:
Many avoid Cabbage because they complain that it makes them gaseous. A pinch of Sugar in Cabbage cuts gas. The health benefits of Cabbage are worth making the effort to enjoy instead of trying to play the avoidance game because of gas.

Cabbage, Turkey Kielbasa and Potatoes

This recipe is my nod to the St. Patrick's Day tradition of Corned Beef and Cabbage. It is at the top of my family's list for comfort food on a snowy or rainy day.

1 head of Cabbage
1 package of Turkey Kielbasa
(for an extra kick can add Halal Hot Turkey Sausage)
5-6 White or Red Potatoes cubed
2 Onions
3 Tablespoons Organic Chicken Better Than Bouillon
1 Tablespoon Vege-Sal
3 Tablespoons Parsley Flakes
2 Tablespoons Caraway Seeds
1 cup water
A pinch of Organic Cane Sugar

-chop Cabbage into 1 inch shreds
-chop Potatoes into 1 inch cubes
-chop Onions into 1 inch diagonals
-cut Turkey Kielbasa into circles
-in a soup pot pour water and Chicken Bouillon, stir until dissolved
-layer bottom of the pot with a lot of Potatoes, some Kielbasa, Cabbage, and Onions

-sparsely sprinkle Vege-Sal, Parsley and Caraway Seeds on the layer
-continue layering and seasoning pattern until all ingredients are used and pot is filled
-cook covered on medium heat
-check for tenderness by turning the pot over and over
-when done mix in Sugar
-serve with hot Cornbread (see recipe)

Asparagus

1 bunch of Asparagus
1 teaspoon Vege-Sal
1 teaspoon Extra Virgin Olive Oil
1 teaspoon Butter
½ fresh squeezed Lemon juice

-steam Asparagus until just tender
-add Olive Oil, Butter, Lemon juice and Vege-Sal to skillet until smoking hot
-toss Asparagus in the mixture until coated and serve immediately

Dr. LaJoyce Brookshire

Parsley Potatoes

4-5 cubed Potatoes
1 Tablespoon Vege-Sal
2 Tablespoons Parsley
2 Tablespoons Butter

-put desired amount of Vege-Sal in water first. Taste test water salty-ness *before* adding potatoes.
-boil potatoes until tender
-drain off water, toss in parsley and butter

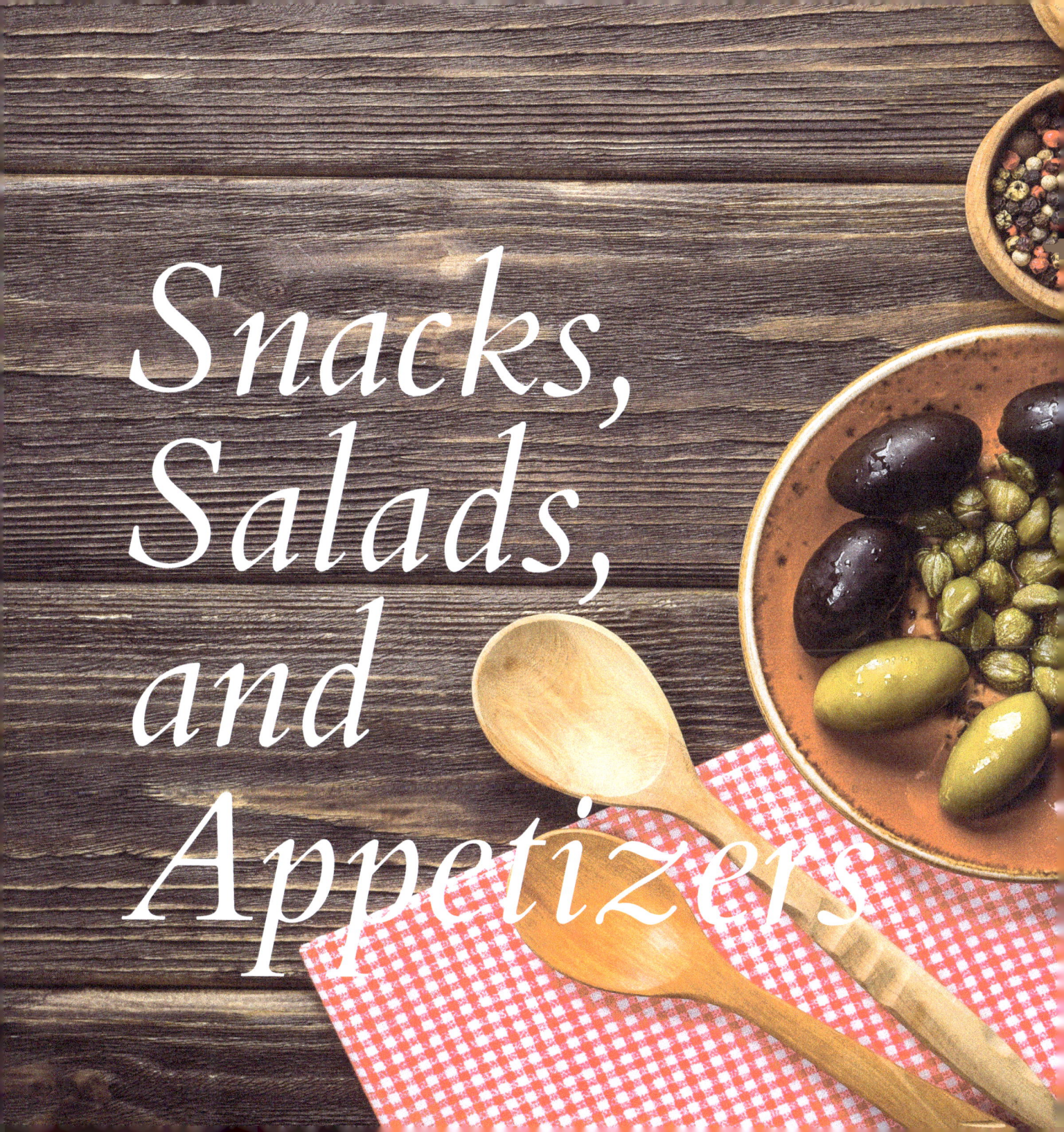

Snacks, Salads, and Appetizers

Dr. LaJoyce Brookshire

Homemade Salad Dressing

Make in a large glass jar:
1 cup Extra-Virgin Olive Oil from First Cold Press
2 cups Bragg's Apple Cider Vinegar
1 Onion chopped
6-7 cloves of Garlic chopped
2 **B**ay Leaves
1 Tablespoon of EVERY herb seasoning in cabinet:
Rosemary, Thyme, Basil, Oregano, Morojam, Parsley, Finest Herbs, Herbs du Provence, Garlic Powder, Onion Powder
a pinch of Cayenne Pepper
Vege-Sal or Himalayan salt to taste
NO Black Pepper!!!

-refrigerate for at least a day and use on salads and marinades for chicken

Fruit Salad

1 whole Pineapple
4 Apples
2 cups Black, Green, or Red Grapes
4 Kiwi
2 cups Strawberries
1 cup Blueberries or Blackberries
2 Pears
1 Lemon

- skin and core Pineapple – chop into cubes and put in bowl
- chop Apples and Pears into cubes and squirt with juice from the Lemon to keep from browning
- skin and slice Kiwi
- slice in Strawberries and fold into the mix
- top off with Blueberries and Grapes

Nutritional Note:
Never mix melons with the any other fruits. Make melon fruit salad with ONLY melons as they do not digest well with other fruits.

Fruit salads are an excellent way to get the recommended 5 servings per day. Having this salad handy takes out the guess-work for a healthy breakfast or snack.

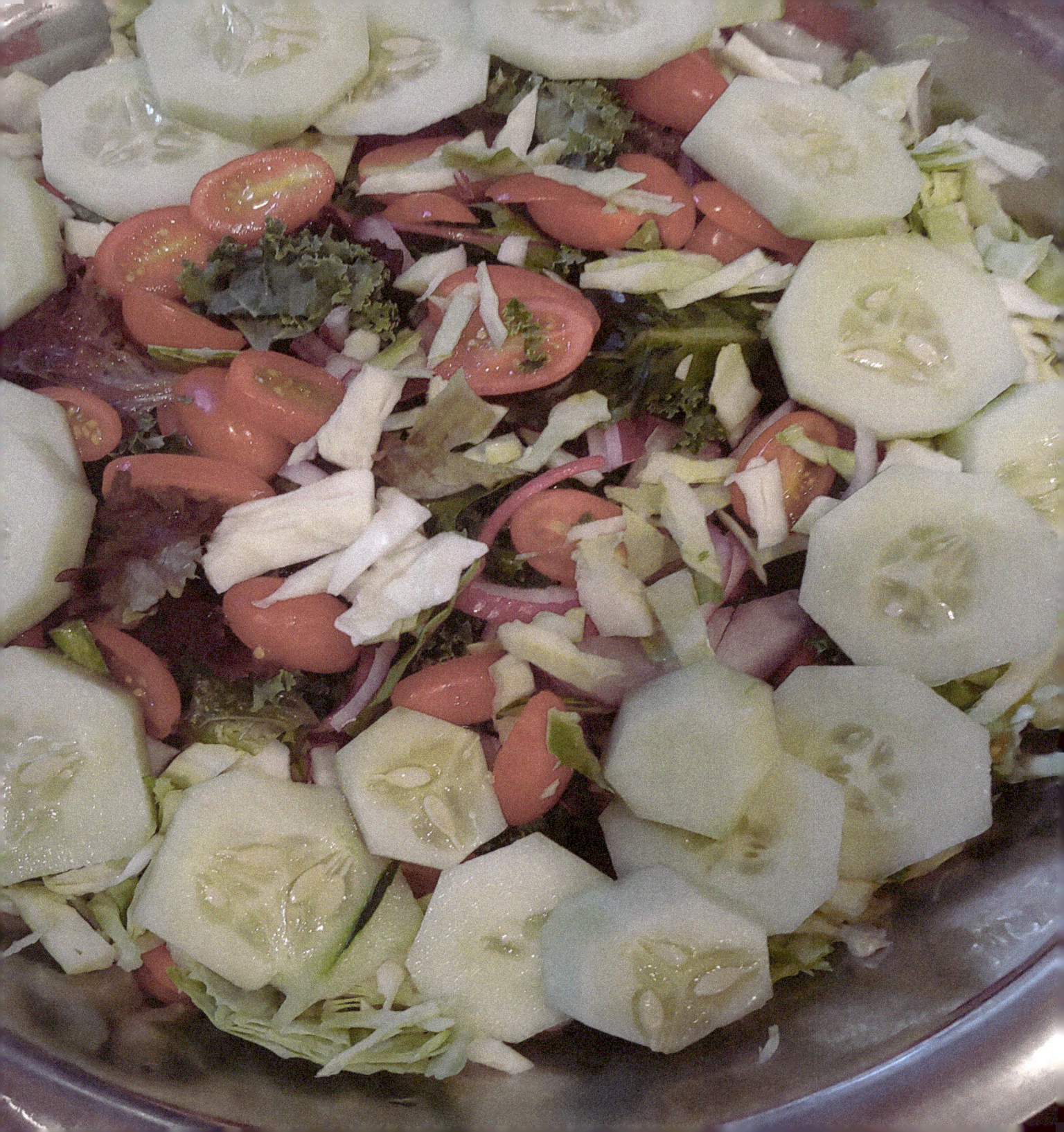

Garbage Salad

Romaine Lettuce
Kale
Red Cabbage
Shredded Carrots
Red Onions
Tomatoes
Cilantro
Cucumber
Broccoli
Avocado
Any kind of crumbly cheese

-layer a salad bowl with each ingredient in the order listed making the next ingredient a little less than the ingredient before it
-scoop salad from the bottom to ensure every plate includes all items
-top with the homemade salad dressing or another healthy favorite

Nutritional Note:
This salad packs a healthy punch with the variety adding fiber and good fats. Making your plate a rainbow becomes a simple task with these ingredients. Fill most of the plate with salad and put other foods around the salad or on top. Use the Homemade Salad Dressing (above) to maximize flavor.

Guacamole

2-3 ripened Avocadoes
2 chopped cloves Garlic
2 sprigs Cilantro
1 small chopped Red Onion
1 chopped Tomato
½ teaspoon Garlic Powder
½ teaspoon Vege-Sal
½ teaspoon Ground Cumin
½ cup Organic Plain Yogurt (Tastes and mixes just like Sour Cream!)
½ juice of fresh Lemon or Lime

-mash Avocadoes in a mixing bowl
-add onion, Tomato, Garlic, and all seasonings and blend well leaving Organic Plain Yogurt until all other ingredients are well mixed
-squeeze in Lemon or Lime and fold-in
-serve with Tortilla Chips and Salsa

Nutritional Note:
The Avocado in Guacamole contribute to healthy fats, vitamins and minerals. Replacing Sour Cream with Organic Plain Yogurt is beneficial due to the probiotics, protein, calcium, magnesium and potassium it contains. Ensure the chip that is dipped is organic! Remember…corn is on the Dirty Dozen list due to pesticides.

Salsa

4 Red and 4 Green Tomatoes
2 Marconi Red Peppers (long sweet peppers)
2 cloves Garlic
1 Jalapeño Pepper (optional)
1 Banana Pepper
1 Onion
1 Green Tomato (Optional)
4-5 sprigs of Cilantro
½ teaspoon Vege-Sal
½ cup Bragg's Apple Cider Vinegar
1 Tablespoon Parsley
Pinch Basil

-mince each ingredient separately in food processor and put in bowl
-add all seasonings and stir
-serve chilled

Caesar Salad a la Martha Stewart

This recipe is a MUST at our annual New Year's Day Get-Down. Each time I make it, I find a way to enhance this salad.

For the Salad:
4 cloves Garlic
3 teaspoons Anchovy Paste
1 teaspoon Vege-Sal
1 teaspoon Cayenne Pepper
1 ½ Tablespoon fresh squeezed Lemon Juice
2 teaspoons Worcestershire Sauce
½ teaspoon Dijon Mustard
1 large Egg yolk
½ cup Extra-Virgin Olive Oil from First Cold Press
2 heads Romaine Lettuce washed and dried
1 ½ cups freshly grated Parmesan or Romano cheese

For the Croutons:
4 Tablespoons butter melted
4 Tablespoons Extra-Virgin Olive Oil
5-6 slices of Multi-Grain, Rye, Pumpernickel or Sprouted bread cubed
1 teaspoon Vege-Sal or Himalayan Salt
½ teaspoon Cayenne Pepper

-make croutons first
-heat oven to 450
-in a skillet combine Butter, Olive Oil, Vege-Sal, and Cayenne until hot
-toss-in the bread cubes until coated evenly
-spread the bread in a single layer on a cookie sheet for about 10 minutes until toasted brown
-set aside until salad is complete

-in a glass jar with a top, blend Garlic and Anchovy Paste until creamy
-whisk in Cayenne, Lemon Juice, Worcestershire Sauce, Dijon Mustard, and Egg Yolk until blended
-add olive oil with a fork
-chop Romaine Leaves and place in a wooden salad bowl with Croutons and Parmesan Cheese
-shake liquid mix on top and toss
-serve immediately
-liquid mix will last 3 days in fridge – shake before each use

Time-Saver Hint:
Double the recipe of the liquid the first time and save for later.

Nachos

1 pound Ground Turkey
4 Tablespoons Cumin
1 Tablespoon Garlic Powder
1 Tablespoon Onion Powder
1 Tablespoon Vege-Sal
1 cup water
1 chopped Onion
2 chopped Tomatoes
1 bunch chopped Scallions
½ can Black Olives chopped
½ can Green Olives chopped
1 cup shredded Mozzarella Cheese
1 cup shredded Cheddar Cheese
Jalapeño Peppers to taste
Pie pan full of plain Organic Corn Tortilla Chips

-brown Turkey meat in skillet
-add Cumin, Garlic and Onion Powder, and Vege-Sal and mix well
-pour in water and cover pot for 15 minutes to simmer
-layer pie pan with Tortilla Chips
-layer ½ cup Mozzarella and ½ cup Cheddar Cheese on top of chips
-put cooked meat on top of cheese and all other ingredients on top of meat
-finish with the other ½ cup of both Mozzarella and Cheddar
-put pan under broiler for 1 minute to melt cheese on top
-serve with additional tortillas, your homemade Salsa, Guacamole, and top with Organic Plain Yogurt

Nutritional Note:
Make a point to have a salad as dinner once a week. To make this appetizer a meal use Romaine Lettuce on the bottom instead of Tortilla Chips. Serve the chips on the side.

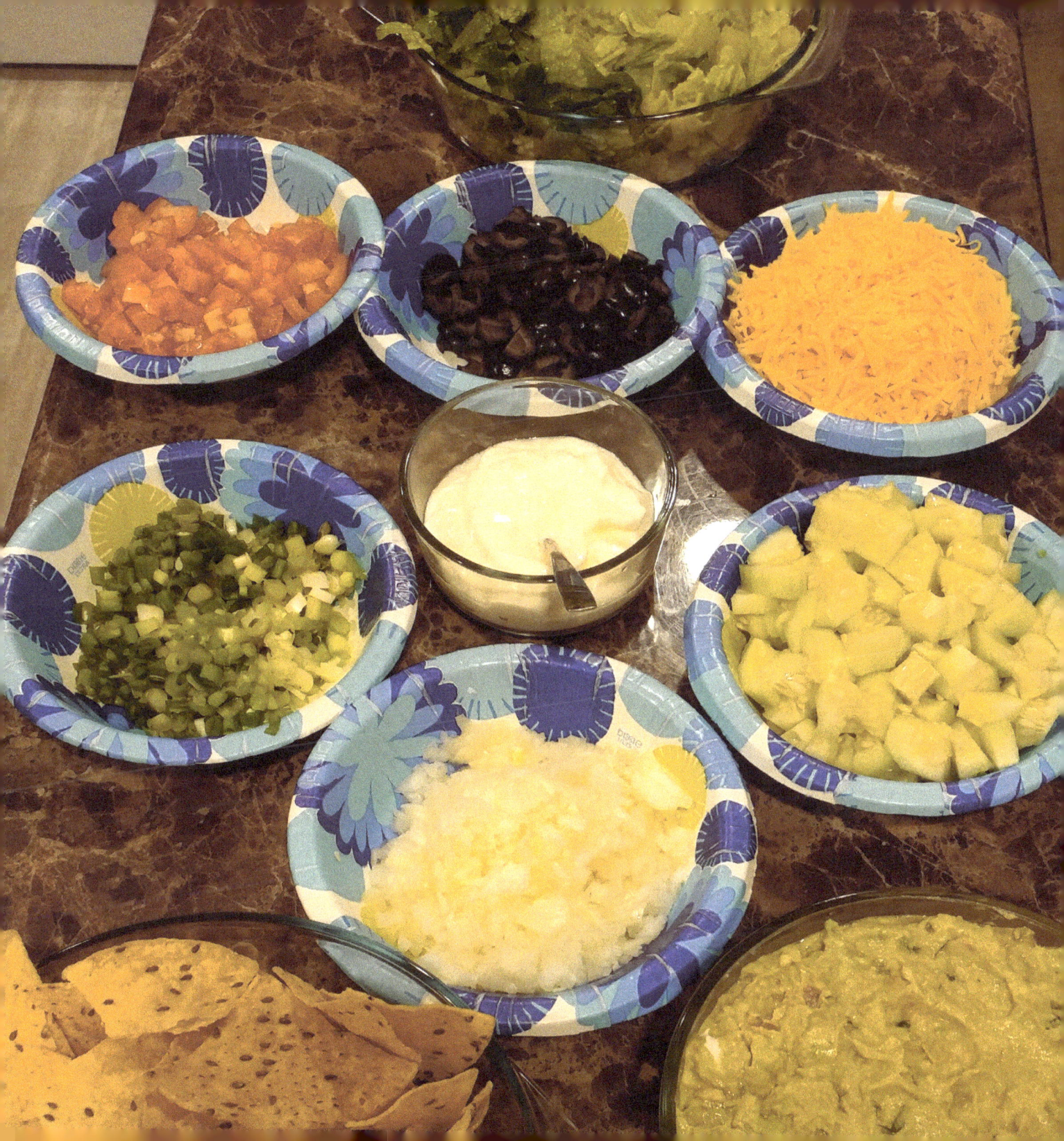

Cole Slaw

1 small head Cabbage
1-2 Carrots
½ Onion
1 cup Miracle Whip
1 Tablespoon Bragg's Apple Cider Vinegar
¼ teaspoon Vege-Sal
¼ teaspoon Celery Seed

-chop Cabbage, Carrots, and Onion into a mixing bowl
-add Miracle Whip, Apple Cider Vinegar, Vege-Sal, Celery Seed
-toss to coat completely
-serve cold

Blue Cheese Cole Slaw

1 small head Cabbage
2 Scallions
1 cup Organic Blue Cheese Dressing

-chop Cabbage and Scallions into a bowl
-coat the Blue Cheese Dressing evenly
-serve cold as a side or on top of a sandwich

Potato Salad

5-6 Red Skin Potatoes
2-3 hard boiled Eggs
2 stalks Celery chopped
1 small Onion chopped
½ cup Green Olives chopped or Capers
1 cup Miracle Whip
A "figure 8" squirt design of Yellow Mustard
¼ teaspoon Celery Salt
¼ teaspoon Vege-Sal

-boil potatoes in the skin* until fork tender
-drain, let cool, peel, and dice
-add Eggs, Celery, Onions, Olives or Capers and mix
-add Miracle Whip, Mustard, Celery Salt, Vege-Sal and mix
-make a day ahead to allow seasonings to meld
*Cooking the potatoes in the skin enhances the flavor of the red potato. The taste is very distinct and pleasant.

snacks, salads, & appetizers

Two-Potato Salad a la The Neeley's

In my house the Food Network is on one TV or another at all times. One of my favorite programs was once "Down Home with The Neely's". While they were lovers of pork, I have had great success re-mixing their dishes.

5-6 Sweet Potatoes peeled and cut into cubes
5-6 White Potatoes peeled and cut into cubes
4 strips crisp-fried Turkey Bacon
1 teaspoon Vege-Sal
4 Scallions finely chopped
2 Celery ribs chopped
1 cup Miracle Whip
2 Tablespoons Creole mustard
1 Tablespoon Herbs du Provence
A few sprigs Cilantro chopped

-fry Turkey Bacon in Olive Oil until crispy on both sides and drain on a paper towel
-cook White Potatoes and Sweet Potatoes in separate saucepans until fork tender
-drain and cool potatoes then add to the same bowl Celery, Miracle Whip, Mustard, Herbs du Provence, Vege-Sal, Cayenne and toss well
-taste test after mixing and add anything additional
-add Cilantro and mix
-garnish with crumbled Turkey Bacon on top

Olives

When my daughter developed a deep, deep love for seasoned Olives of any kind, there was not an Olive Bar that she would pass without filling-up a container. At $8.99 per pound in most stores I knew I had to find a way to duplicate the savory seasoned Olives we all love at a fraction of the cost and without any preservatives. I even bottle in fancy glass jars and give as gifts.

All Olives should be pitted:
2 Cans Black Olives
2 Jars Kalamata Olives
2 Jars Spanish Olives (Manzanilla)
2 Mason Jars 16 oz
Sliced Garlic
Garlic Powder
Coarse Sea Salt
Thyme
Basil
Rosemary
Oregano
Crushed Red Pepper
Extra Virgin Olive Oil from First Cold-Press
Organic Red Wine Vinegar
(Use the quantity of seasoning to your taste. We like them bold, intense and savory. Start with a little seasoning, and then add a lot as desired. This is my technique.)

-drain the juice off of all of the Olives, rinse thoroughly and allow to air-dry a bit
-in a large mixing bowl place all of the Olives
-shake the Coarse Sea Salt over the bowl of Olives
-slice fresh Garlic and liberally shake Garlic Powder, Thyme, Basil, Rosemary, Oregano, Crushed Red Pepper

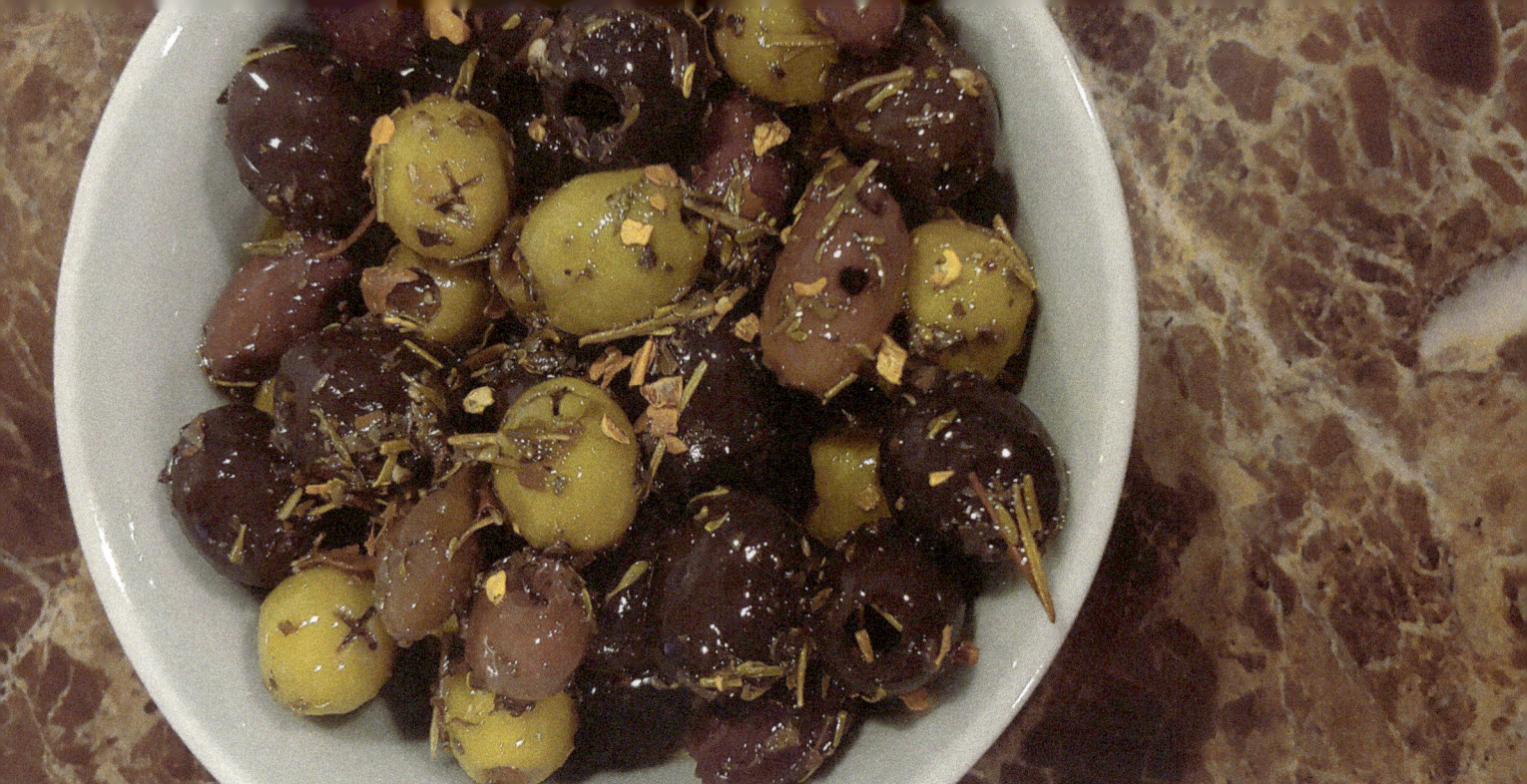

- mix all gently with a large spoon and fill the Mason Jars just under the rim
- fill the jars with 1/4 cup of Extra Virgin Olive and then fill the jar with Red Wine Vinegar to the top of the Olives
- close the jar and shake to blend the Olive Oil and Red Wine Vinegar well
- turn jar upside down on counter to allow the seasoning to saturate all the way to the top
- the next day turn the jar to normal position and continue to allow all seasoning to meld
- put in fridge for longevity
- allow to set at room temperature before serving
- try different variations and NEVER pay $8.99 per pound again!

TIP: Reserve the jars from the store, soak off the labels, and when you want to give your Olives to someone you love, a jar is handy!

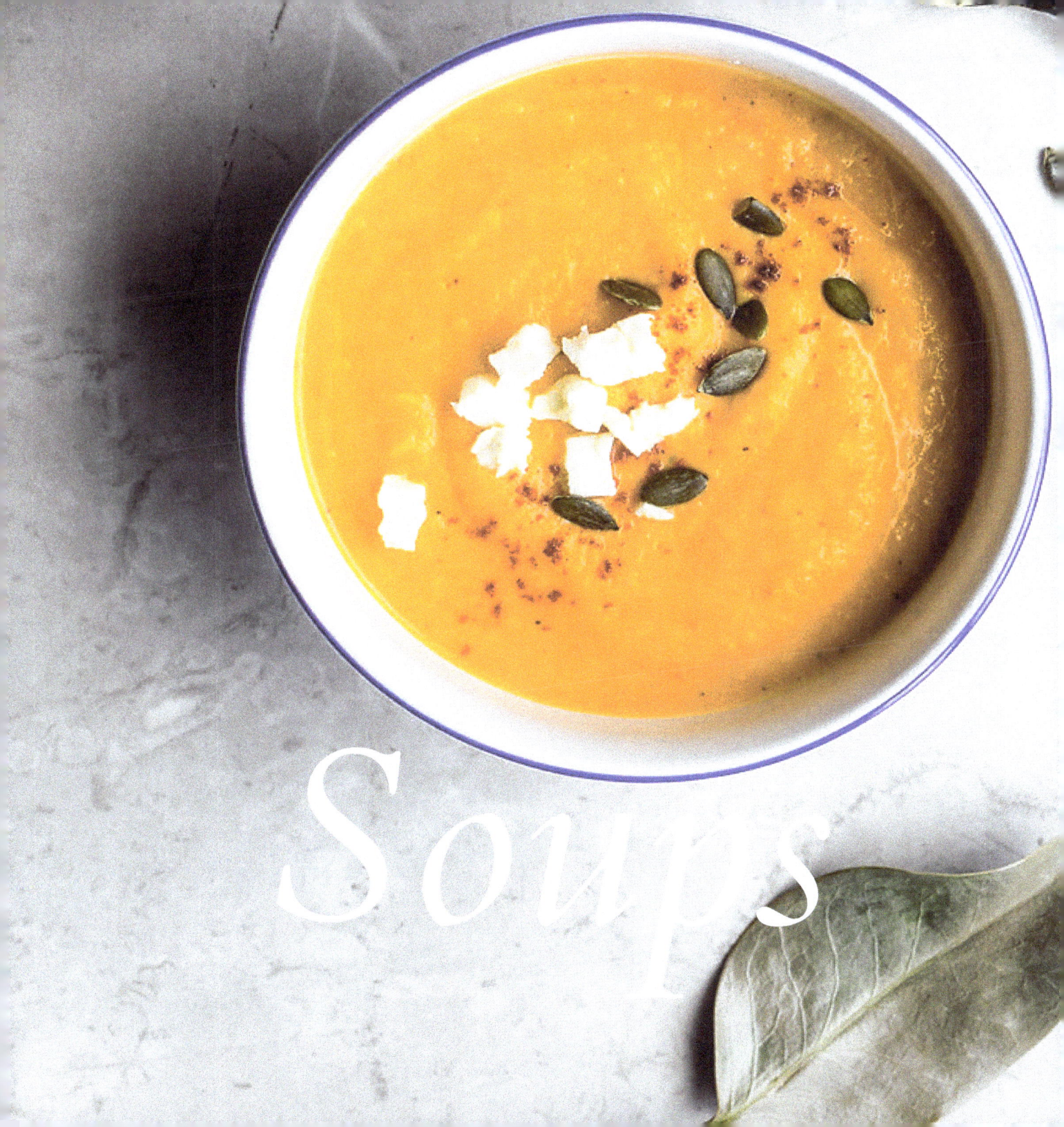

Soups

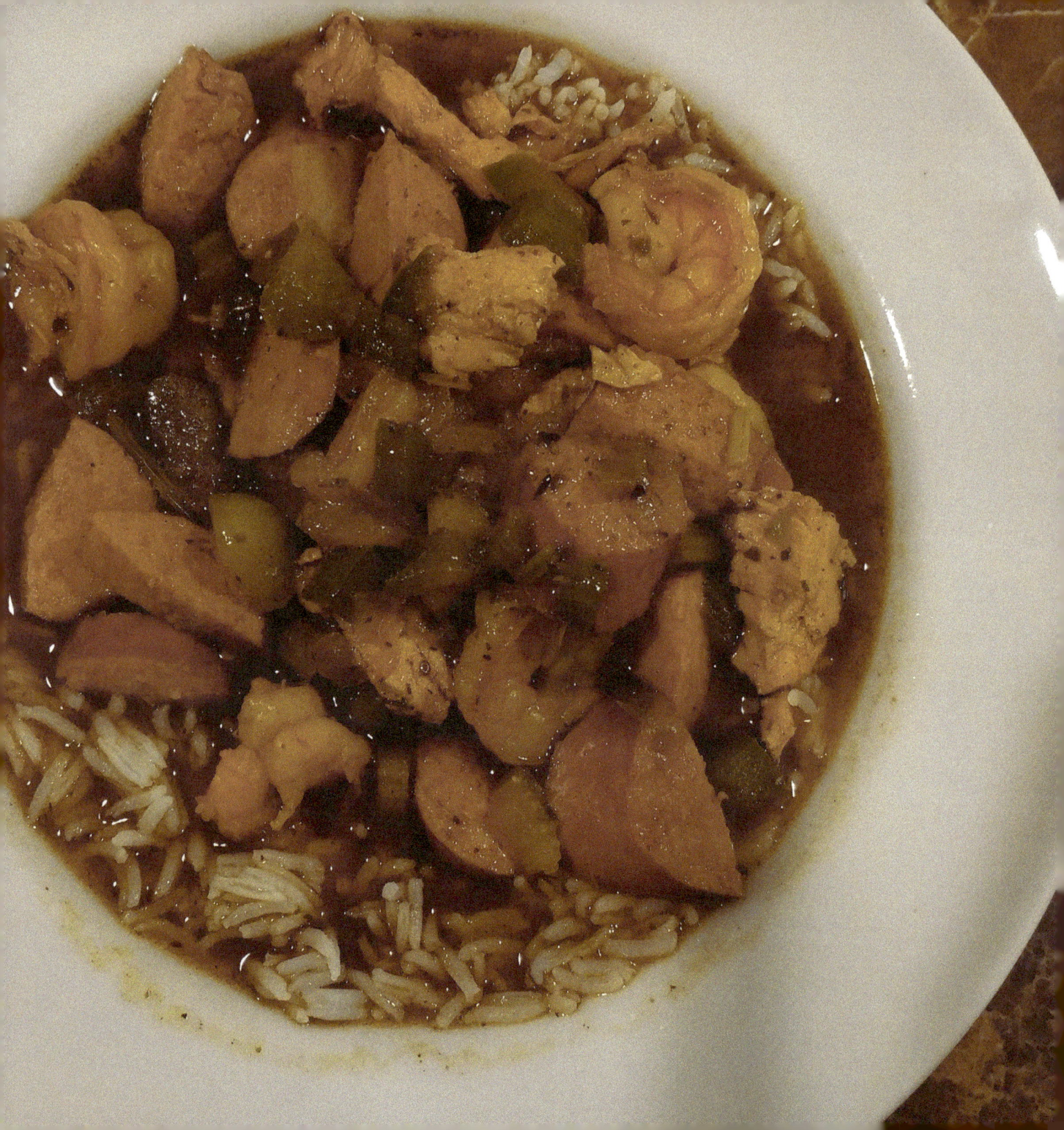

Gumbo a la "Mommie Jo"

As a native of Louisiana, my Mommie developed into a fantastic cook albeit strictly textbook. Gumbo is one of the dishes she is begged to make for any occasion. It has been varied much from the original and my recipe has been given her official stamp of approval, "You've got it down pat, girl!" The labor intensity is worth every moment to create this masterpiece.

8 cups water (6 from Shrimp shells, 2 from Turkey Kielbasa)
1 stick Butter
4 Tablespoons Unbleached Flour
3 Onions chopped
2 Green Peppers chopped
2 bunches Scallions chopped
6 cloves Garlic
4 Bay Leaves
2 Tablespoons Garlic Powder
2 Tablespoons Onion Powder
1 Tablespoon Thyme
1 teaspoon Sweet Basil
4 Tablespoons Organic Chicken Better Than Bouillon
2 Tablespoons Vege-Sal
2 Tablespoons Worcestershire Sauce
¼ cup Hot Sauce
2 pounds Turkey Kielbasa (replaces pork smoked sausage)

2 pounds shell-on green Shrimp (raw shrimp in the shell)
4 boneless skinless Chicken Breast
1 pound Crab Legs (optional)

- in a large pot, boil Chicken breasts until done, drain stock into a glass jar and let cool (save chicken stock for fridge to use at another time)
- clean and shell Shrimp - put in a bowl for later and put shells in a pot with enough water to cover at least 2 inches over shells
- boil shells on low heat until pink
- drain off 6 cups of the shell water into a large bowl
- cut Turkey Kielbasa into round pieces and put into a pot to cover at least 2 inches over the sausage and boil
- drain off 2-4 cups of the sausage water into a measuring cup
- melt butter in heavy soup pot and stir in flour
- constantly stir the flour butter mix over low heat for about 15 minutes until flour turns a deep brown – this process is called making a Roux
- add 6 cups Shrimp water, 2 cups Sausage water, Garlic, Garlic Powder, Onion Powder, Bay Leaves, Chicken Bouillon, Thyme, Sweet Basil, or Sauce, Worcestershire Sauce, and Vege-Sal to the Roux
- cover pot and cook 10 minutes on low to develop flavor
- shred Chicken breasts on the grain so that there are a heap of Chicken shreds
- add Chicken, Sausage rounds, onions, Scallions, Green Peppers and cook 15 minutes
- serve after pot has had a chance to sit at least 1 hour over hot Basmati Rice in large bowls with multi-grain crackers.
- Gumbo tastes its best the day after it is cooked

Split Pea Soup

An essential item for all kitchens is the Crock Pot. This utensil is the most awesome time saver! I keep my Crock Pot on the counter all year long and use it every Sunday. After church we enter the house to a soup that is ready to eat as the aroma greets us at the door.

6-8 cups of water in a Crock Pot
1 bag of dried Split Peas
2 Bay Leaves
2 Tablespoons Better Than Bouillon Organic Chicken Flavored Paste
1 Tablespoon Vege-Sal
1 Tablespoon Garlic Powder
1 Tablespoon Onion Powder
1 Onion chopped
2 Garlic Cloves chopped
2 Tablespoons Parsley

-put hot water into crock pot and turn on high with bouillon, Bay Leaves, Vege-Sal, Garlic powder, Onion powder, Onion, Garlic, and Parsley
-rinse Peas in a strainer and discard any imperfect peas or rocks
-put Peas in Crock Pot and set to high for 3-4 hours*
-4 hours cook time on high will yield a smooth Pea soup
-3 hours cook time will still have some in-tact peas

Dr. LaJoyce Brookshire

Chicken Noodle Soup

4 skinless chicken breasts
Soup pot with 8 cups water
2 bay leaves
2-4 Tablespoons Organic Chicken Better Than Bouillon
2 Tablespoons garlic powder
2 Tablespoons onion powder
1 Tablespoon Vege-Sal
½ Tablespoon each of Thyme, Rosemary, Sweet Basil
2 Celery stalks chopped
2 Onions chopped
1 Green Pepper chopped
4 Garlic cloves chopped
1 cup Cabbage shredded
5 Carrots diced
2 cups Kale shredded
½ bag vegetable pasta noodles (optional)
*for an occasional Tomato Based soup, add 1 jar of your own Tomato Sauce or Newman's Tomato Basil Sauce

-boil Chicken breasts in water with Bay Leaves until done, scoop out Chicken and let cool
-to the stock add Better Than Bouillon, Garlic Powder, Onion Powder, Vege-Sal, Thyme, Rosemary, Sweet Basil, Celery, Green Pepper, Garlic cloves, Cabbage, and simmer 15 minutes

-meanwhile, shred Chicken on the grain so that there are a heap of Chicken shreds and mix into pot

Kitchen Warriors 101: Homemade Healthy

-after 10 minutes add Carrots and Kale and bring to a rolling boil
-at the boiling peak, add the Noodles dunking them into the soup, and turn off the pot but leave on the stove
-serve with homemade bread

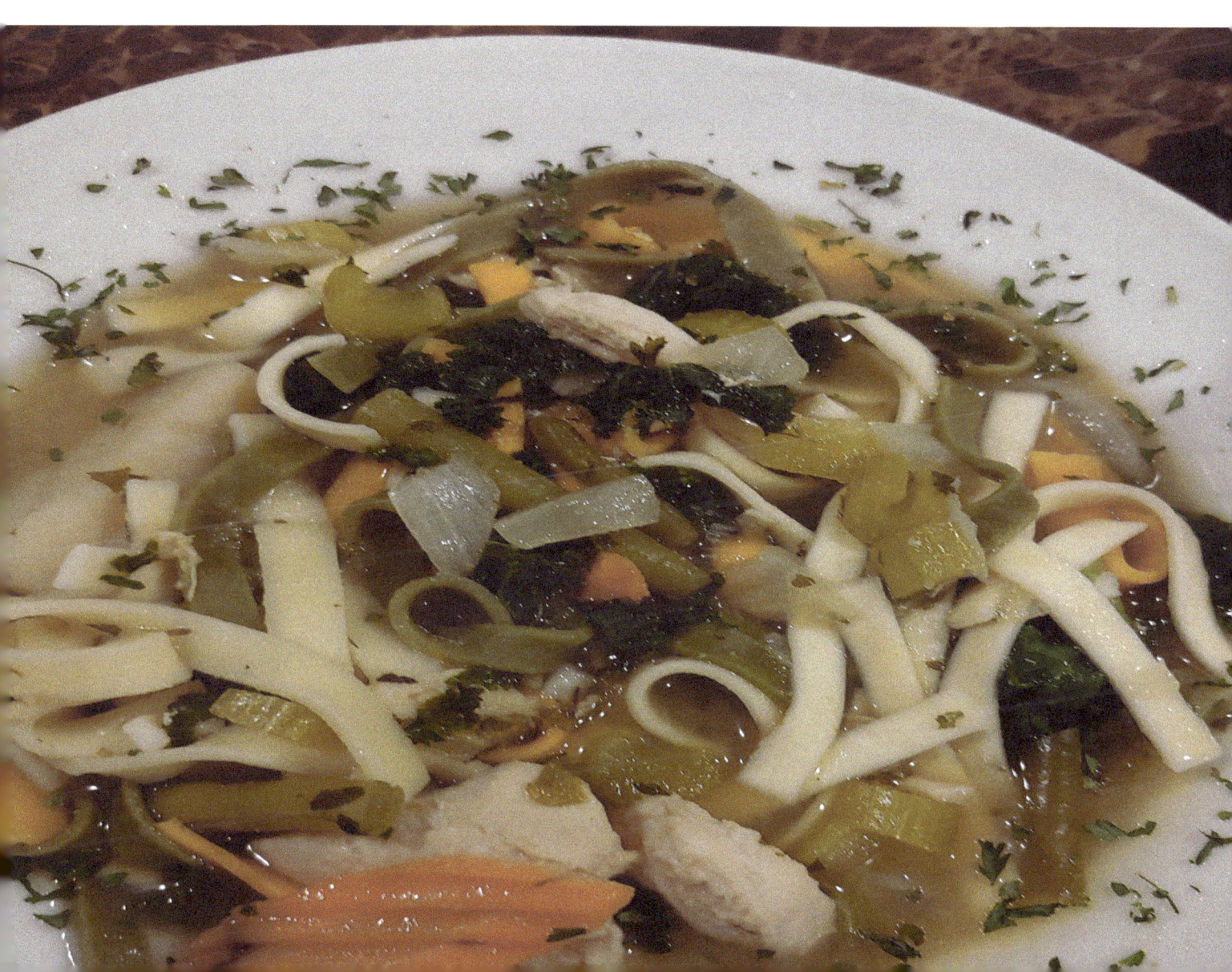

Black Bean Soup

6-8 cups hot water in Crock Pot
2 Bay Leaves
2 Tablespoons Organic Chicken Better Than Bouillon
1 Tablespoon Vege-Sal
1 Tablespoon Garlic powder
1 Tablespoon Onion powder
1 Onion chopped
1 Celery rib chopped
2 Garlic cloves chopped
2 Tablespoons Parsley
2 Tablespoons Cumin
1 teaspoon Cayenne Pepper

-put hot water into Crock Pot and turn on high with bouillon, Bay Leaves, Vege-Sal, Garlic powder, Onion powder, Onion, Celery, Garlic, Cumin, Cayenne, and Parsley
-rinse Beans in a strainer and discard any imperfect beans or rocks
-put Beans in Crock Pot and set on high 4 hours or low 6-7 hours

Red Beans and Rice

1 package dried Red Beans
2 Bay Leaves
2 Tablespoons Organic Chicken Better Than Bouillon
1 Tablespoon Vege-Sal
1 Tablespoon Garlic powder
1 Tablespoon Onion powder
1 Onion chopped
2 Garlic cloves chopped
2 Tablespoons Parsley

-fill soup pot with 8-10 cups hot water and bring to a rapid boil with all ingredients except beans
-taste test the water for desired seasoning levels
-rinse Beans in a strainer and pick out rocks and imperfections
-pour beans into pot and bring to a fast boil
-turn down to low heat and allow to cook for 2-3 hours or until desired tenderness is reached (if water boils out and beans are not cooked, in another pot boil hot water to add)
-for a thick gravy, when beans are just done, dump a tray of ice cubes into the pot and this will thicken-up the broth
-serve over rice and with hot cornbread

Dr. LaJoyce Brookshire

Award Winning Slammin' Savory Organic Turkey Chilli

My Chilli has always been a friend and family favorite. I decided to put it to the test in 2012 at a local Chilli Cook-Off at the Shawnee Mountain Annual Rodeo. I was the only "Kitchen Cook" amidst 12 restaurants and I won Second Place! I will add that this recipe it filled with love and nutrients which satisfies any tummy on any day.

2 pounds ground Turkey
1 large can dark Red Kidney Beans
1 large can light Red Kidney Beans
2 cans Black Beans
2 Onions chopped
4 Celery ribs chopped
2 Green Peppers chopped
4 Bay Leaves
6 cloves Garlic chopped
4 cans crushed Tomatoes
2 large cans tomato paste + 2 cans water -or- defrost homemade Tomato sauce in necessary quantity
3 Tablespoons Hot Chilli Powder (or Mild Chilli Powder)
2 Tablespoons Vege-Sal
4 Tablespoons Garlic powder
4 Tablespoons Onion powder

8 Tablespoons Cumin
2 Tablespoons Celery salt
1 Tablespoon Cayenne Pepper
2 Tablespoons Oregano
2 Tablespoons Sweet Basil
4 Tablespoons Parsley
1 Tablespoon dried Minced Onion
¼ cup Extra Virgin Olive Oil

- in a large soup pot warm Olive Oil until hot and add ground Turkey. Cook until completely browned
- season the Turkey with all of the seasonings except Bay Leaves and blend
- add Tomato sauces and pastes with water and Bay Leaves. Simmer for 15-20 minutes
- add all of the rinsed Beans to the pot
- cover and simmer until contents begins to bubble – stir frequently
- add the Onions, Celery, Green Pepper last so there will be crunch to the veggies
- most excellent the day after cooking

Coconut Milk Soup

This Thai soup has been a favorite of mine for years. When the restaurant started adding ingredients I did not like, it was time to learn to make it myself.

2 cans Coconut Milk
2 Tablespoons Chicken Better Than Bouillon
2 Tablespoons Lemongrass Paste or fresh Lemongrass
Chopped Green Onions, Orange Peppers, Red Peppers, Broccoli, Bok Choy, Snow Peas
Pinch of Parsley

-heat Coconut Milk on low heat
-stir in Better Than Bouillon until dissolved
-stir in Lemongrass Paste until dissolved or add in fresh Lemongrass
-when milk begins to lightly boil add in all chopped ingredients
-serve immediately into bowls over brown Basmati Rice

Low Country Boil

I first experienced this dish in Savannah, Georgia on our annual Girls Trip with my college friends Debbie and Faye. It was originally made with pork sausage. This is my variation which includes the addition of a little this and a little that…

Large Heavy Soup Pot
10 cups water
2 packages No Nitrite/No Nitrate Turkey Kielbasa sliced
3 pounds Jumbo Shell-on green (raw) Wild-Caught Shrimp in the shell
2 pounds Wild-Caught King Crab Legs
4-6 ears fresh Organic Corn halved or Organic Frozen Corn Halves
6-8 Red Potatoes in the skin halved
6 whole cloves Garlic
10 Bay Leaves
3 Onions halved
1 handful fresh Italian Parsley chopped
3 Tablespoons Old Bay Seasoning
2 Tablespoons Oregano
1 Tablespoon Garlic powder
1 Tablespoon Onion powder
1 Tablespoon Allspice
1 Tablespoon Dill
1 Tablespoon Rosemary
1 teaspoon Cayenne Pepper

Dr. LaJoyce Brookshire

-fill pot with water adding whole Bay Leaves, Garlic, Garlic powder, Onions, Onion powder, Oregano, Allspice, Old Bay Seasoning, Dill, Rosemary, chopped Parsley, Cayenne Pepper, and Turkey Kielbasa cut in 1-inch angle slices
-when water comes to a boil add King Crab Legs, and Red Potatoes
-just as Potatoes are fork tender add the Shrimp and Corn cover, and turn off the stove

-melt butter for dipping
-roll-up sleeves and enjoy!!

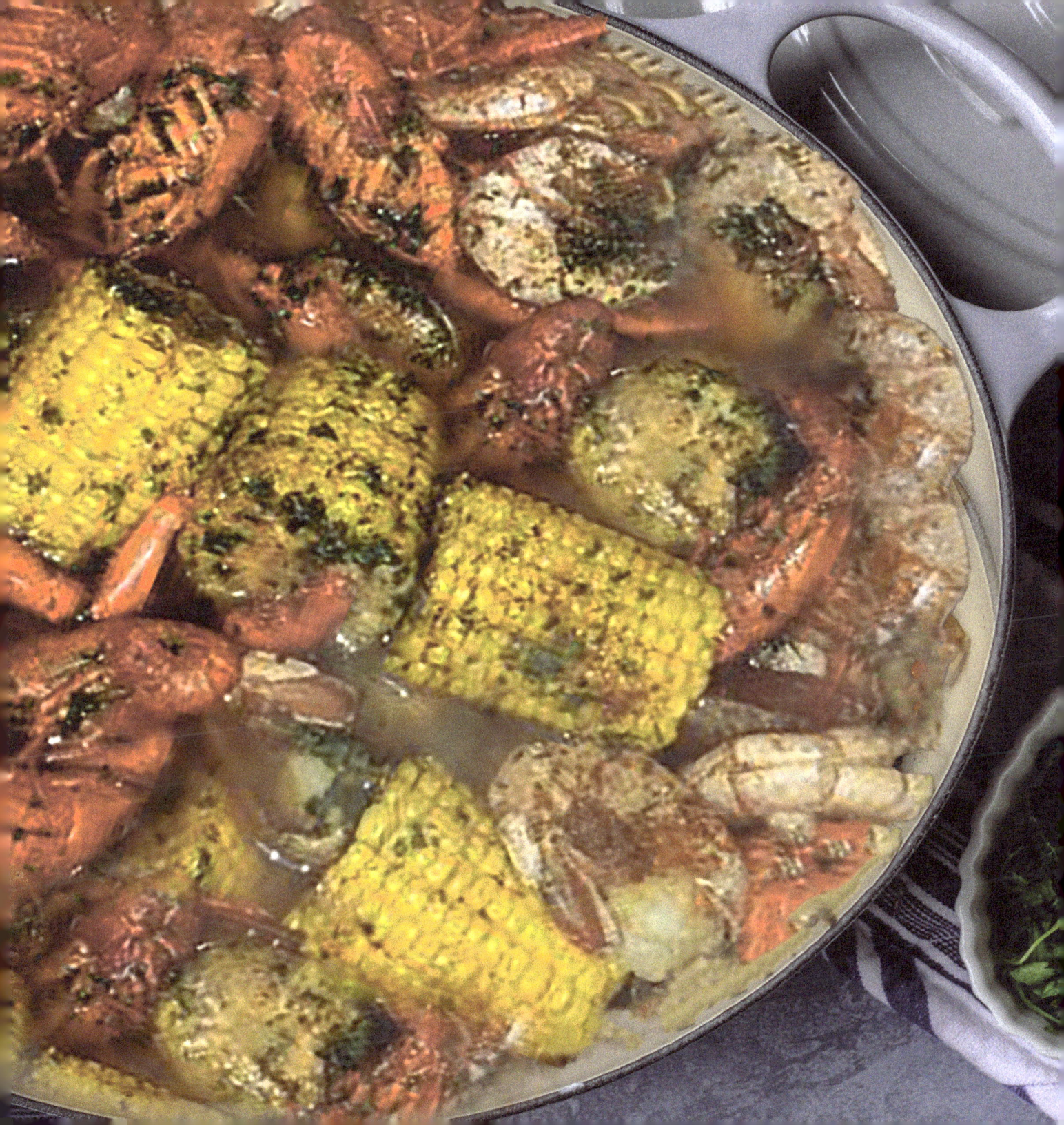

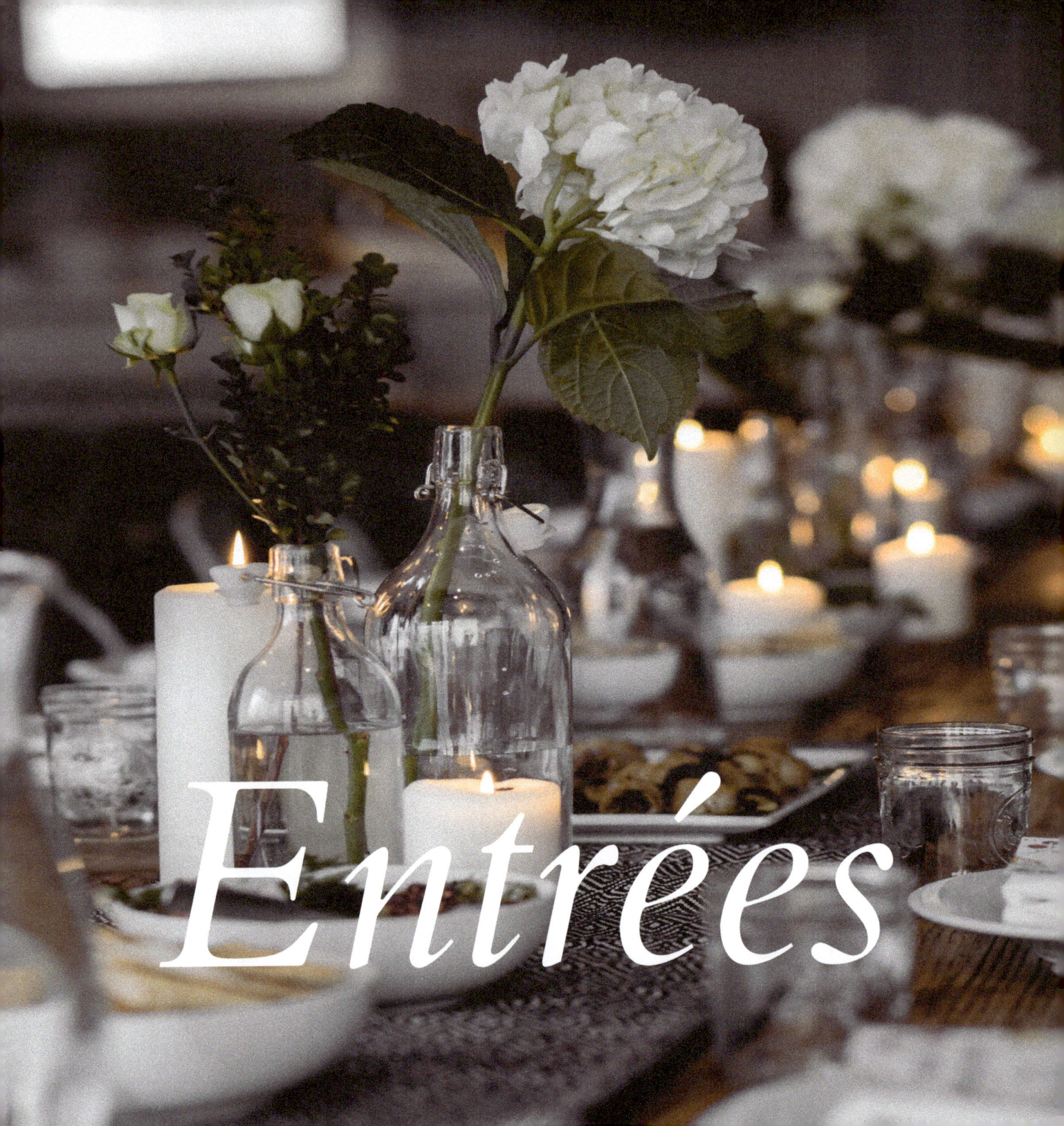

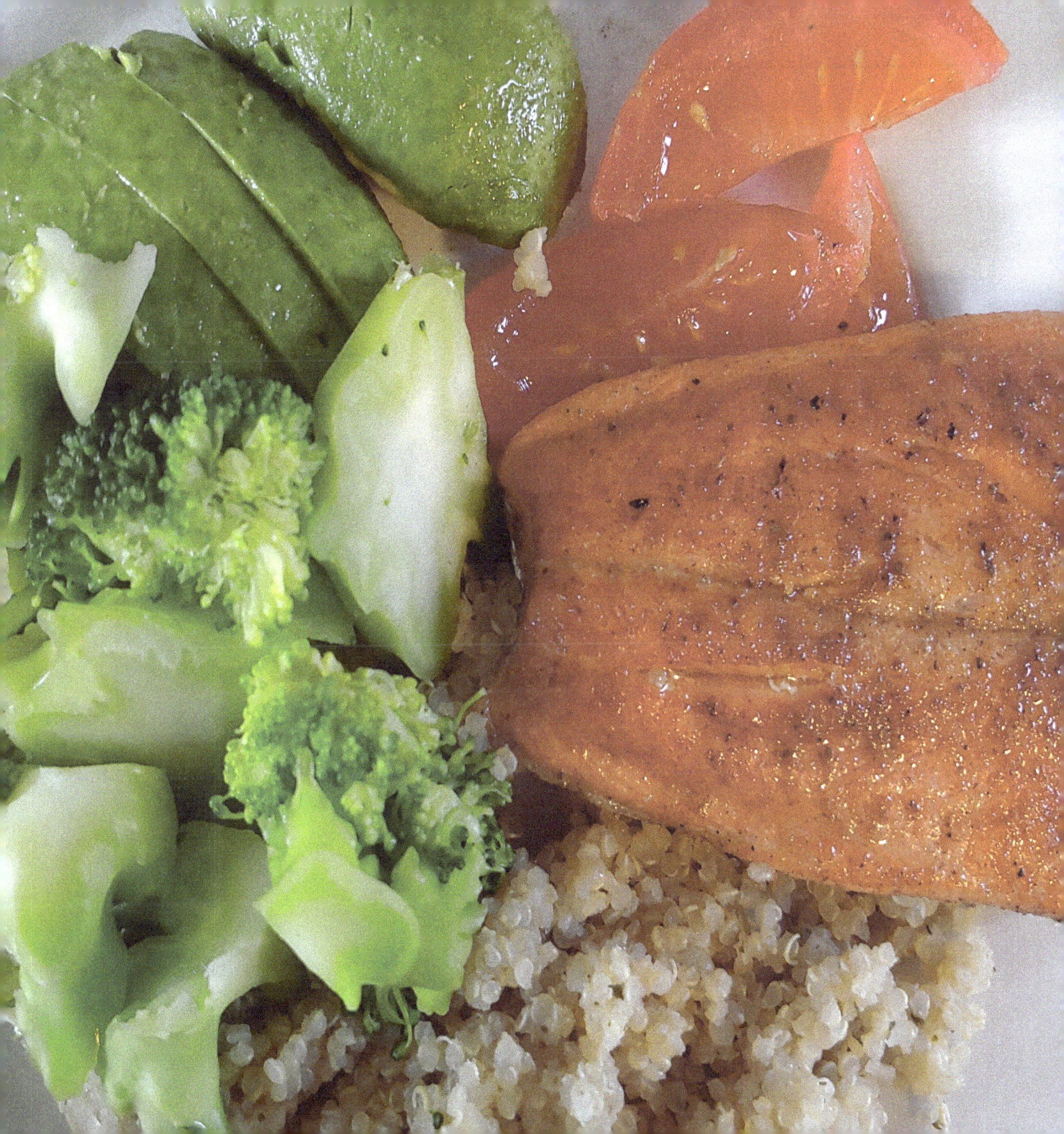

Dr. LaJoyce Brookshire

Pan Seared Salmon

4 pieces wild-caught Salmon
1 teaspoon Vege-Sal
1/2 teaspoon Dill
½ teaspoon Parsley
1 pat of Butter for the top of each piece
Extra Virgin Olive Oil

-heat olive oil to hot enough to coat the bottom of skillet then add Salmon, Vege-Sal, and Dill
-when Salmon begins to turn light pink place a pat of butter on top and garnish with dried parsley
-serve on top of Asparagus, Broccoli Rabe, or Salad

Broiled Salmon with Lemon Butter Sauce, Tomatoes and Capers

4 pieces wild-caught Salmon
1 teaspoon Vege-Sal
1 teaspoon Herbs du Provence
½ teaspoon Parsley
1 pat of Butter for the top of each piece
Extra Virgin Olive Oil

Sauce:
3 lemons squeezed
1 Tablespoon Lemon Zest
1 stick Butter
2 Tomatoes chopped
1 cup Capers

- grease each Salmon piece with Olive Oil and arrange in a well-greased broiler pan
- season with Vege-Sal, Herbs du Provence, Parsley
- using the fine side of a cheese grater, shred Lemon rind until 1 Tablespoon of Zest is accumulated.
- place Salmon in broiler
- in a skillet melt Butter, adding Zest, Tomatoes, Capers, and Parsley
- remove Salmon when done
- serve fillets with a spoonful of sauce on top of each piece on a bed of bitter greens of choice

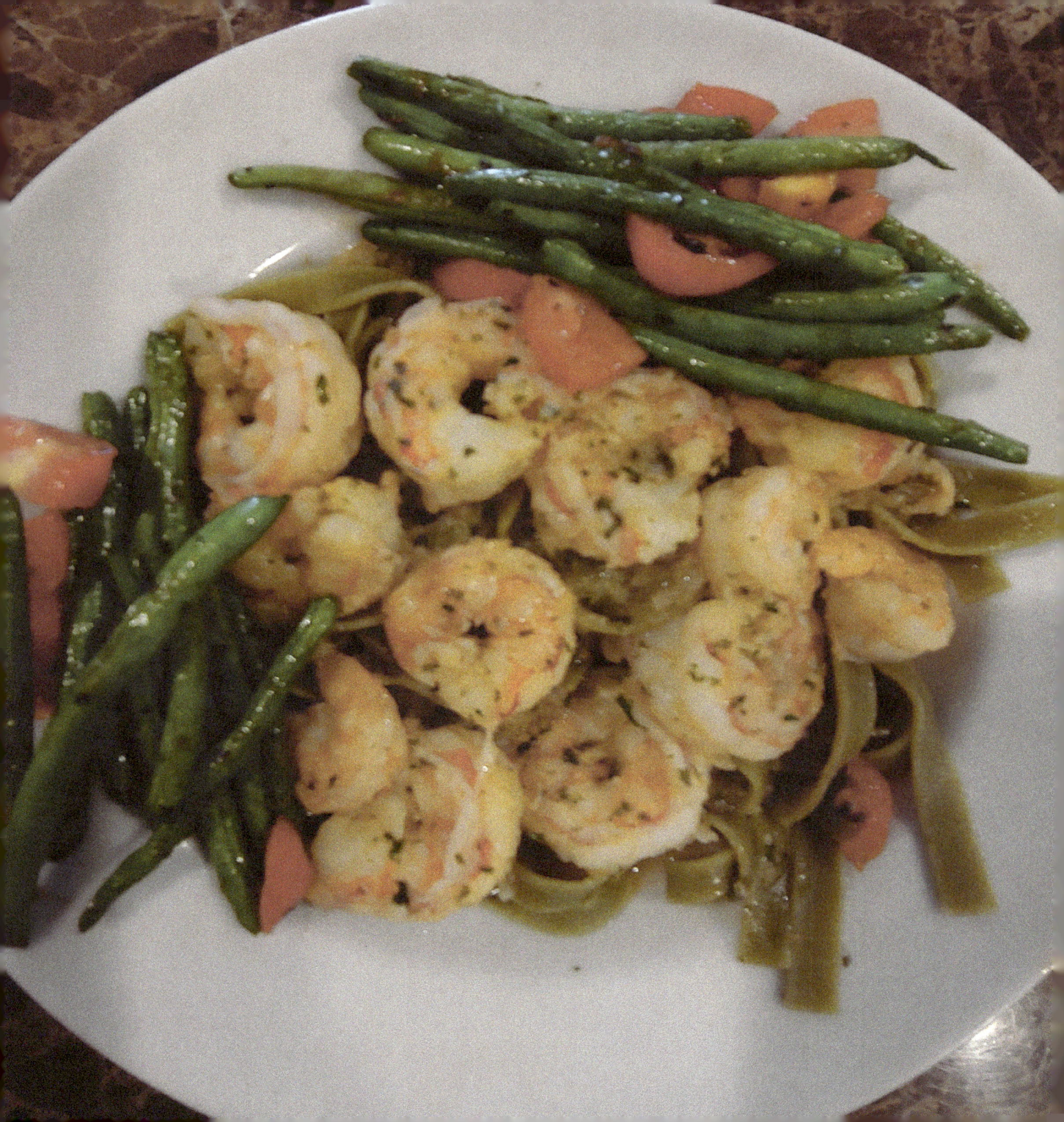

Shrimp and Scallop Scampi

This family favorite is one of the most requested plates in my arsenal. My darling mentee Karu Daniels who named me "The Good Doctor" in the first-place squeals with glee when I make this dish for his birthday annually. Once in the kitchen of my dear girlfriend Robbin who just had to have a lesson of this dish, she has nicknamed it simply, "One Stick of Butter". Keeping these ingredients on hand can make you look like a hero in a pinch.

1 stick Butter
¼ cup Extra Virgin Olive Oil
1 ½ Onion chopped
1 cup Garlic chopped
½ Tablespoon Vege-Sal
1 Tablespoon Garlic powder
1 Tablespoon Onion powder
2 Tablespoons Parsley
1 pound jumbo shell-on green (raw) Shrimp with
1 pound Scallops
½ cup Shrimp shell water
1 cup Capers
2 Lemons squeezed
1 Tablespoon Lemon Zest
1 package Angel Hair pasta

A few shakes of hot sauce
-peel Shrimp and put the shells in a saucepan completely covering the shells
-boil shells until they turn pink
-drain off ½ cup Shrimp water for Scampi sauce and pour the balance of Shrimp into a saucepan to cook pasta
-add water to Shrimp water for pasta, Vege-Sal salt to taste and add a few drops of Olive Oil
-melt Butter in a large skillet and add Garlic, Onion, Vege-Sal, Garlic powder, Onion powder, and Parsley stirring to mix
-as the sauce thickens add the shrimp water and allow to boil
-add Angel Hair pasta to boiling salted water
-add Scallops to butter mix and cook covered for 5 minutes
-add Shrimp, Capers, and Zest continually tossing to coat
-drain Pasta and place in bowls
-pour Lemon juice into the cooked pot and blend
-spoon Scampi onto waiting pasta bowls

Salmon Croquettes

1 can wild Alaskan pink or red Salmon
2 Eggs beaten
½ Onion chopped
1 teaspoon Garlic powder
¼ teaspoon Onion powder
¼ teaspoon Vege-Sal
Panko Crispy Bread Crumbs (test quantity)
Extra Virgin Olive Oil

- drain water from Salmon can, dump into a bowl and mash with a fork including the bones
- beat in eggs, onion, garlic powder, onion powder, Vege-Sal
- after blending start adding Panko Crumbs until the mixture will successfully hold the shape of a patty
- pour ¼ inch olive oil in heavy skillet over medium heat
- scoop 1 Tablespoon of Salmon mixture into hand and press to make a patty
- put patty on a spatchula and slide into hot oil
- flip ONLY when oil side has browned
- drain on a paper-towel lined cookie sheet
- Croquettes should be crispy – use regular bread crumbs to avoid the crispy or bake

Nutritional Note:
The bones in canned Salmon is loaded with Calcium. The bones are very soft and crumble easily making it easy to mix while preparing and you never notice while chewing. Use a high-quality Wild-Caught Red or Pink Salmon canned to reap the benefit of the good fat from Omega-3.

Dr. LaJoyce Brookshire

Foil Baked Haddock or Cod

1 pound Haddock or Cod (can be frozen
½ of a Green, Red, Orange, and Yellow Pepper sliced
1 Onion sliced
1 teaspoon Vege-Sal
½ teaspoon Garlic powder
½ teaspoon Herbs du Provence
1 teaspoon Parsley
Extra Virgin Olive oil

-preheat oven to 450
-line a baking dish with foil large enough to hang over the sides, slice onion and place on greased foil
-wash and dry fresh Fish, (wash frozen fish) and oil-up each piece back and front then arrange on top of onions and some of the Pepper mix
-season with Vege-Sal, garlic powder, Herbs du Provence, and parsley
-load on the remaining Peppers and seal the tops and sides of the Fish with foil
-the top piece of foil should meet the bottom piece and roll tightly until sealed all around
-bake about 20 minutes
-serve with steamed Broccoli or sautéed Spinach

Crispy Oven-Baked Italian Chicken

4 drumsticks
4 thighs
4 chicken breasts
2 cups Homemade Dressing(see recipe) or Italian dressing
1 teaspoon Onion powder
1 teaspoon Garlic powder
1 teaspoon Basil
1 teaspoon Thyme
1 teaspoon Rosemary

-lower rack to mid-oven and preheat to 550 degrees or on its highest heat setting – NOT broil
-pour 1 cup of Homemade Dressing or Italian Dressing into a baking dish
-arrange Chicken onto dressing skin side down onto dish
-pour 1 cup of dressing on top of Chicken (can use more if needed)
-put in fridge to marinate overnight or at least 2 hours
-in a foil lined pan arrange Chicken skin side up – reserve marinade
-sprinkle all seasonings onto Chicken and spoon marinade on each piece
-put in oven and cook on 550 for ONLY 20 minutes
-then lower temperature to 375 to continue cooking
-the chicken breasts will be done first so rescue them in about 10 minutes
-take out chicken when the outside is dark brown indicating it being well-done and with a crispy coating

Dr. LaJoyce Brookshire

Fried Chicken Wings

I fry chicken only once a year which is at our New Year's Day Get-Down. Friends gather in my kitchen for this favorite and they are even crazy enough to eat them right out of the oil. For them, no cooling period is necessary.

12 whole Chicken Wings
Extra-Virgin Olive oil
2 cups Unbleached flour
2 Eggs beaten
1 Tablespoon Vege-Sal
1 Tablespoon Onion powder
1 Tablespoon Garlic powder
½ Tablespoon Sage
1 Tablespoon Parsley
1 teaspoon Dry Mustard
1 teaspoon Cayenne
1 large heavy Soup Pot or Cast Iron Pot

-wash and pat dry Chicken Wings with a paper towel
-put Chicken in a bowl with the Eggs
-fill a large pot fill ½ full with Olive Oil and turn on medium heat
-in a bowl mix Flour and all seasonings then pour into the bowl with Chicken and Eggs
-toss around well to fully coat Chicken with the seasoned Flour
-the Chicken will be pasty
-drop 4-5 wings at a time into the hot oil
-they will turn golden brown and float when done

Whole Stewed Chicken a la Aunt Mabel

The matriarch in our family was Aunt Mabel who died at 83. She was once a cook for a New York City hospital and catered functions from scratch. This woman could COOK!! When she died, her mind was still really sharp and she could whip out a recipe from memory like she cooked it yesterday. See…I keep saying you are what you eat…

1 whole Chicken washed and dried
½ cup Garlic chopped
2 Onions chopped
3-4 Celery ribs chopped
1 bunch Scallions
5-6 Carrots slivered
6-7 Red Potatoes
1 cup Bragg's Liquid Aminos (tastes EXACTLY like soy sauce)
1 Tablespoon Parsley
5 cups water
Extra Virgin Olive Oil

-preheat oven to 550 degrees
-cook Chicken in oven for 20 minutes until browned all over
-meanwhile chop all fresh items
-once Chicken has browned pour in Bragg's Liquid Aminos and water
-add all chopped Veggies and cover for about 1 hour over low heat,
-when done add Carrots and Red Potatoes
-serve over Rice or Noodles

Dr. LaJoyce Brookshire

Smothered Chicken

1 whole Chicken cut up or favorite pieces and seasoned
1 cup unbleached Flour
1 Tablespoon Vege-Sal
1 Tablespoon Garlic Powder
1 Tablespoon Onion Powder
1 Tablespoon Ground Thyme
2 Onions slivered
Extra Virgin Olive Oil

-heat enough Olive Oil in bottom of skillet to coat
-put all seasonings in Flour
-dredge Chicken pieces in seasoned Flour
-place in hot oil and brown on all sides
-remove to paper towel
-add 1 slivered onion to the remaining chicken grease and sauté
-in a bowl mix 2 cups water + 1 cup flour to make gravy
-when well blended pour into the skillet with onion and oil
-continually stir until gravy turns brown
-return chicken skillet with gravy
-place 1 slivered onion on top of chicken
-cover pot and cook on low until fork tender

Broccoli Rabe with Vegetable Noodles

1 bunch Broccoli Rabe
1 bag Vegetable Noodles
4-5 Garlic cloves chopped
1 cup Locatelli cheese shredded
½ cup Extra Virgin Olive Oil
1 tablespoon Vege-Sal
¼ cup water reserve from Noodles

-use a steamer that has a bottom section
-fill pot with water, Vege-Sal, and a dip of Olive Oil
-chop Broccoli Rabe and place in the steamer portion of the pot and place on top
-add bag of Noodles to the boiling water, return steamer portion to the top of pot and cover
-chop Garlic
-Noodles will be al dente in 10-12 minutes
-remove Broccoli Rabe in steamer and drain Noodles
-in the base of the pot heat Olive Oil and Garlic
-when Garlic turns brown add Broccoli Rabe, Noodle water reserve, and sauté
-add Noodles last with Locatelli cheese and mix all ingredients well

Smoked Turkey Glazed with Orange Marmalade and Dijon Mustard

So…this is one of those recipes that I have no idea of how much to use. I just sprinkle with all of the seasonings inside and out until the turkey is completely covered

1 smoked organic Turkey
2 Apples sliced
2 Celery Ribs
Vege-Sal
Sage
Thyme
Parsley
Onion powder
Garlic powder
1 jar Orange Marmelade
1 cup Dijon Mustang

-wash Turkey completely and dry with paper towels
-sprinkle seasonings on Turkey until covered
-stuff inside of Turkey cavity with Celery and Apples peeled and halved
-put 1 cup water in the bottom of the roasting pan
-cook covered on 300 for one hour less than indicated based on weight
-mix Orange Marmalade and 1 cup of Dijon Mustard together
-remove Turkey from oven and brush on the glaze thickly
-return Turkey back to oven and cook uncovered at least 1 more hour, until brown

Nutritional Note:
If finding an Organic Smoked Turkey is a challenge, be adventurous and smoke a regular Turkey yourself in a smoker. Your family will never want a regular Turkey again.

Turkey Italian Sausage

Finding quality Turkey products can be a laborious process. I have discovered a local Turkey farmer where I get a variety of products made fresh from organically grown Turkey.

8 Turkey Hot Italian Sausages
1 Red Pepper sliced
1 Orange Pepper sliced
1 Green Pepper sliced
1 Yellow Pepper sliced
1 Onion sliced
¼ cup Extra Virgin Olive Oil
½ cup water

-in a skillet place water and Oil in bottom
-arrange the Sausage so they are not touching
-cook on medium heat and cover
-turn occasionally to brown do not let water boil out, add more when needed
-when Sausage is brown on all sides toss in all sliced Peppers and Onion and cover
-serve over hot Brown Rice

Dr. LaJoyce Brookshire

Turkey Burgers

1 pound ground Turkey – not the white meat
1 Onion chopped
1 Green Pepper chopped
½ Tablespoon Vege-Sal
Extra Virgin Olive Oil
2 packages Vegetarian Brown Gravy Mix (optional)
(this is a gravy mix is quickie short cut that tastes JUST like homemade)

-mix all ingredients in a bowl
-scoop out 1 tablespoon of mix and make into a ball
-in 425 degree oven- press the burgers onto a greased cookie sheet and cook until done
-or-
 on the stove top- press out Turkey balls into patties and put into hot greased skillet

-in a sauce pan cook Gravy mix
-add Turkey Patties to Gravy with sliced Onion and cover pot to simmer
-serve over hot Brown Rice, Cous Cous, or Wild Rice

Bar-B-Que Turkey Meatloaf

1 pound ground Turkey
1 Onion chopped
1 Green Pepper chopped
½ Tablespoon Garlic Powder
1 Tablespoon Yellow Mustard
½ cup Bar-B-Que Sauce
Extra Virgin Olive Oil
½ cup **B**ar-B-Que sauce for topping

-mix all ingredients by hand in a bowl
-in a add Turkey mix to a greased casserole dish and shape into a loaf
-bake at 350 for 45 minutes
-pour last of the Bar-B-Que Sauce over the top and allow to bake 15-20 minutes…Perfection!

Turkey Meat Balls with Brown Gravy a la Wylene

My dear friend Wylene has the assignment of making her Signature Dish which are the Turkey Meatballs for our New Year's Day Get-Down. I learned how to master and then RE-master her recipe which we enjoy regularly. Wylene has her homemade gravy down to a science that is sopping good. My gravy skills need help and this is one of the places where I cheat with Vegetarian Brown Gravy that is as good as homemade and has no additives or preservatives.

entrées

1 pound ground Turkey
1 Green Pepper chopped
1 Onion chopped
½ teaspoon Cumin
½ cup Worchester Sauce
4 packages Vegetarian Brown Gravy

-mix all ingredients in a large bowl
-heat oven to 350 - prepare 2 well greased, foiled lined cookie sheets
-scoop 1 Tablespoon of Turkey mix and roll into a ball arranging on cookie sheets ¼ inch apart
-bake in oven until light brown
-in a large soup pot make Gravy
-add meatballs to the gravy when done and cook on top stove over medium heat until boiling

Egg Foo Young

I first tried to make this favorite of mine on my own when:
1. I got tired of getting the Chinese take-out home and my Egg Foo Young would be burnt.
2. I got tired of the restaurant not having what I consider the 'main' ingredient…Bean Sprouts.

4 organic Eggs
1 bunch Scallions (tops only)
½ Onion slivered
½ cup of any other vegetable (optional)

½ cup Bean Sprouts (the round white ones)
1 package Hain Vegetarian Brown Gravy

-prepare gravy in a saucepan and leave on the side
-heat oil in the skillet
-meanwhile chop veggies, put in pan, and sauté
-beat eggs and pour evenly on top of vegetables
-sprinkle Vege-Sal, parsley, and sprouts on top
-cook slowly to allow egg to get done
-fold egg in half when the top is no longer runny
-pour gravy over the eggs and serve over hot Brown Basmati Rice

Nutritional Note:
Bean Sprouts are the most Alkaline food on the planet. When striving for perfect health, alkalinity is our best bet. A healthy body thrives when it is alkaline and no disease can live in it. A sick body is guaranteed to be acidic. Bean Sprouts are a nutritious way to eat your way to good health. Try them in Stir-Fry, Salads, and Soups.

Zoodles with Turkey Meat Sauce

Zucchini (2 healthy sized) or 1 pre-Spiraled package
1 pound ground Turkey
3 jars of homemade sauce or Newman's Tomato Basil Sauce
1 Onion
2 Celery ribs chopped
5 Garlic cloves chopped
1 each Green, Red, Yellow, and Orange Pepper
1 Tablespoon Vege-Sal
1 Tablespoon Onion powder
1 Tablespoon Garlic powder
2 leaves fresh Basil chopped or torn
1 Tablespoon Oregano
2 Tablespoons Parsley
Pinch of Cayenne Pepper
Extra Virgin Olive Oil
Shaved Parmesan Cheese

-Wash and dry Zucchini and Spiralize into Zoodles or wash and pat dry the pre-packaged Zoodles
*TIP – salt water first to desired level so that the Zoodles will absorb while cooking. It is much more difficult to salt once done.
-when sauce begins to boil, add onions, Celery, and all colored Peppers, Cayenne pepper and blend well
-when Zoodles have cooked to al dente remove from heat, drain, and fill bowls putting Turkey sauce on top
-brown ground Turkey in soup pot with Olive Oil
-when Turkey begins to brown, add, Garlic, Vege-Sal, Onion powder, Garlic powder, Basil, Oregano, and Parsley – mix together well

Kitchen Warriors 101: Homemade Healthy

- add Tomato sauce and cover pot on low heat
- fill another saucepan with water and desired amount of Vege-Sal and a drizzle of Olive Oil to prevent sticking
- serve with shaved Parmesan Cheese

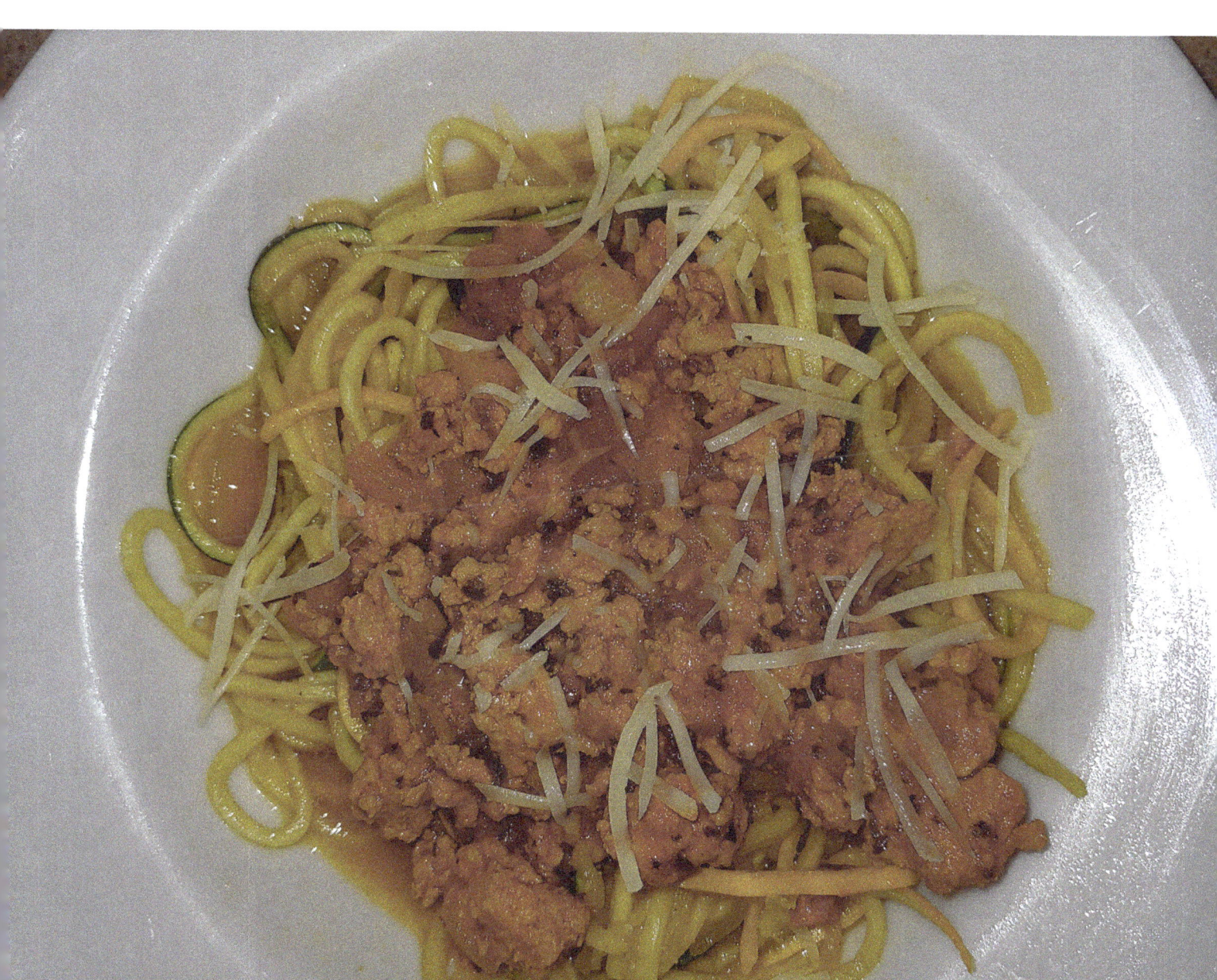

Seafood Spaghetti

I created this delight when in college and I was running for Miss Alpha Phi Alpha. I served this dish to the fraternity and watched them eat bowl after bowl until the roasting pan was empty. I won first runner-up because of this meal… Scrumptious!

1 pound Shrimp raw in the shell
1 pound Scallops
1 pound Crabmeat shelled
3 jars of homemade sauce or Newman's Tomato Basil Sauce
1 Onion
2 Celery ribs chopped
5 Garlic cloves chopped
1 each Green, Red, Yellow, and Orange Pepper
1 can Black Olives halved
1 Tablespoon Vege-Sal
1 Tablespoon Onion powder
1 Tablespoon Garlic powder
2 leaves fresh Basil chopped or torn
1 Tablespoon Oregano
2 Tablespoons Parsley
Pinch of Cayenne Pepper
Extra Virgin Olive Oil
Shaved Parmesan Cheese

- peel Shrimp and put shells in a saucepan with enough water to cover top of shells
- cook shells until turned pink – reserve shell water
- with sauce in soup pot add Garlic, Vege-Sal, Onion powder, Garlic powder, Basil, Oregano, and Parsley – mix together well
- add shell water, cover and simmer 15-20 mins
- fill another saucepan with water and desired amount of Vege-Sal and a drizzle of Olive Oil to prevent sticking

*TIP – salt water first to desired level so that the pasta will absorb while cooking. It is much more difficult to salt once done.

- when sauce begins to boil, add Seafood, Onions, Celery, all colored Peppers, Black Olives, and Cayenne Pepper blending well cover and turn off heat
- Seafood will cook on its own due to the heat of the pot – allow the sauce to meld the flavors
- when Spaghetti has cooked to al dente remove from heat, drain, and fill bowls putting Seafood sauce on top
- serve with shaved Parmesan Cheese, Garbage Salad, hot Mozzarella Cheesy Garlic Bread (See recipes)

Dr. LaJoyce Brookshire

Spinach Fettuccini Alfredo

1 box Spinach Fettuccini pasta
1 quart heavy Whipping Cream or Half and Half
1 teaspoon Vege-Sal
½ Onion chopped
¼ teaspoon Nutmeg
½ stick Butter
1 cup Broccoli, or Shrimp, or Chicken
Pinch of Cayenne Pepper
1 cup shaved Parmesan Cheese

-boil Spinach Fettuccini in Vege-Sal salted water
-in a sauce pan, melt Butter, chopped Onion, Nutmeg and blend
-add heavy Whipping Cream stirring constantly until it thickens
-add shaved Parmesan Cheese to cream mix and stir
-drain Fettuccini noodles and combine with creamy mix (can add Broccoli, Shrimp, or Chicken at this time)

Eggplant Parmesan

My sister Alicia LOVES this dish and I have to admit I do too. She wants me make a ready quantity for her freezer any time I am in Chicago. I have to admit that it is awesome tasting and really healthy.

2 large Eggplant with skin in ½ inch slices
3 eggs
2-3 cups plain Bread Crumbs
3 jars of Homemade Sauce or Newman's Tomato Basil Sauce
1 Onion
2 stalks Celery Chopped
5 cloves Garlic
1 each Green, Red, Yellow, and Orange Pepper
1 Tablespoon Vege-Sal
1 Tablespoon Onion powder
1 Tablespoon Garlic powder
2 leaves fresh Basil chopped or torn
1 Tablespoon Oregano
2 Tablespoons Parsley
Pinch of Cayenne Pepper
3 cups Fresh Mozzarella Cheese
2 cups Parmesan Cheese
Extra Virgin Olive Oil

-in a large sauccpan put Tomato Sauce, Garlic, Vege-Sal, Onion powder, Garlic powder, Basil, Oregano, and Parsley – mix together well and cover pot on low heat

-line a large cookie sheet with Parchment Paper
-cut Eggplant in half length-wise and turn the cut-side down toward cutting board
-cut Eggplant from base to the stem in ½ inch slices and dunk in Egg
-dredge in Bread Crumbs and place on Parchment Paper then place in the oven and bake on 400 until bread crumbs are brown
-when all of the Eggplant is browned, arrange Eggplant in the bottom of a well-greased
casserole dish until the bottom is covered
-layer Tomato sauce over Eggplant, then Mozarella over Tomato Sauce, then Parmesan over Mozzarella then another layer of Eggplant until cheese is covered
-repeat process to the top of the casserole dish
-finish off with sauce and cheeses on top
-bake at 350 until bubbly

* TIP – this dish freezes well. Sometimes, instead of making an entire full casserole dish, I will make the Eggplant rounds larger and prepare each round with its own sauce and cheese. This way I can grab one or two out of the freezer and have Eggplant anytime.

Nutritional Note:
Use Eggplant with the skin-on for the best nutritional punch as it is loaded with vitamins and minerals. Eggplant is also great roasted in the oven or grilled. Drizzle with a little Extra Virgin Olive Oil first.

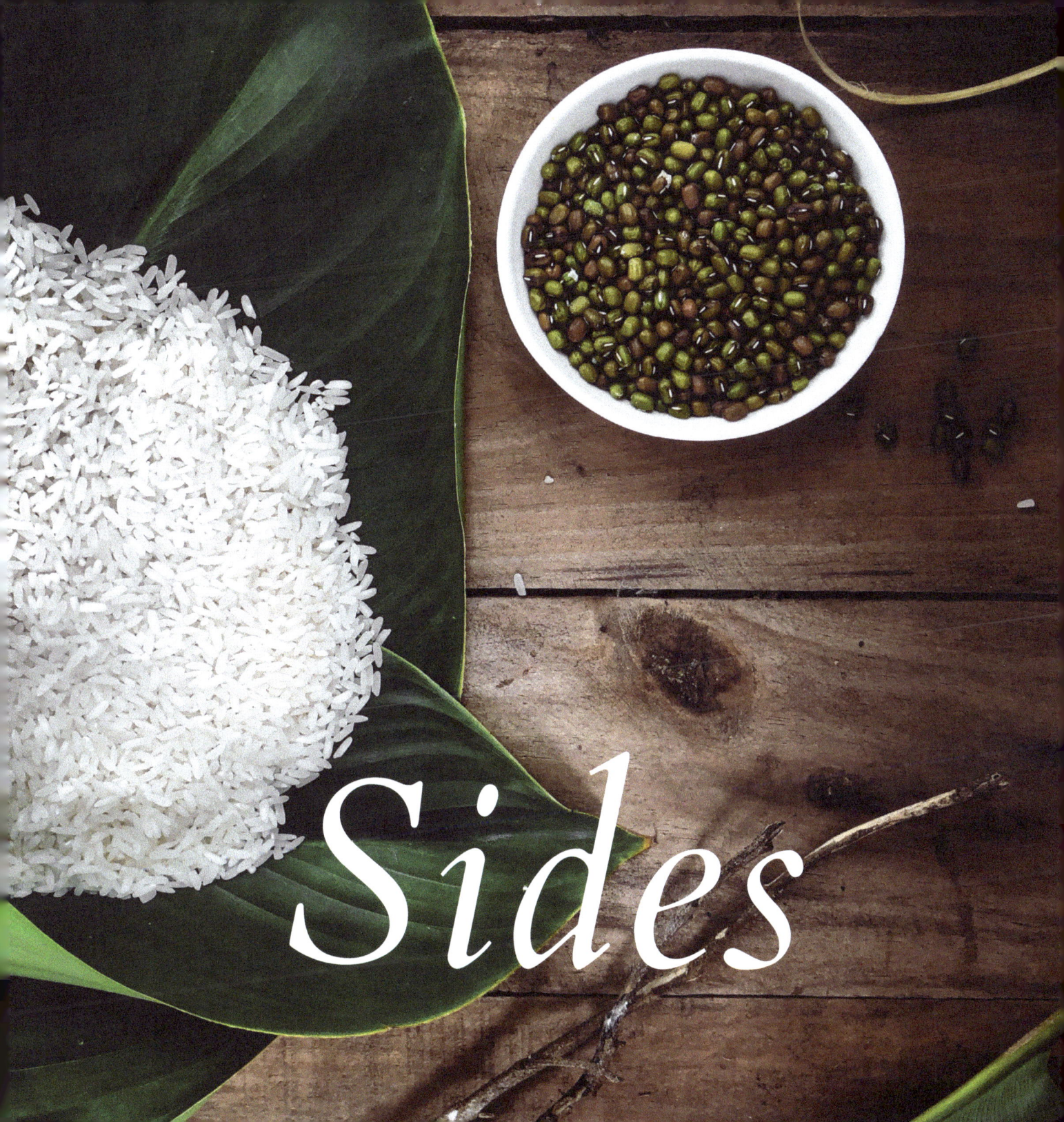

Sides

Dr. LaJoyce Brookshire

Macaroni and Cheese

1 pound box of elbow Macaroni (vegetable, whole wheat, or gluten free)
8 oz White Cheddar Cheese shredded or cubed
1 ½ cup Milk
1 Tablespoon Dry Mustard
½ Onion chopped
½ stick Butter
3 Tablespoons Flour

-boil salted water and add Macaroni
-Make a Roux: in a saucepan melt Butter with chopped Onions
-add Dry Mustard
-add Flour one tablespoon at a time (the mix should be creamy, if too pasty add more butter one teaspoon at a time until creamy)
-pour in Milk and stir until Roux thickens
-add cubed or shredded Cheese and stir until melted
-drain cooked Macaroni and put in a greased casserole dish
(reserve 1 cup or more of Macaroni to ensure there is enough Cheese sauce to coat all of the Macaroni)
-pour Cheese sauce over Macaroni and toss to blend well – the mix should be really creamy
-can eat as is or bake in oven
-To Bake: beat 2 eggs over mixture and blend-in
-bake on 425 until bubbly brown

Potato Salad

7-9 Red Skin Potatoes
Vege-Sal to taste
2 ribs Celery chopped
1 small Onion chopped
2 Eggs diced
10-12 Green Olives halved
1 cup Miracle Whip

- salt water until it is well-salted with Vege-Sal
- boil Red Skin Potatoes in jackets
- chop all veggies and eggs
- when potatoes cool, gently peel away skin
- dice potatoes and add all ingredients and blend

Nutritional Note:
To increase fiber content keep skins on the potatoes. A boiled Red Potato with the skin peeled away leaves a very distinct taste and they are loaded with phytonutrients.

Green Rice

My favorite rice's are Basmati in Brown, White, Light Brown, varieties and traditional Brown Rice. Basmati Rice is not processed making it a healthier choice. It is a long grain – making it sturdier than other types - and it is very aromatic. I enjoy making varied rice dishes because they can go from being a side dish to an entrée when served with a salad and veggies.

1 cup favorite Basmati rice variety
2 cups water
1 chopped Green Pepper
½ cup Parsley
2 Tablespoons Organic Chicken Better Than Bouillon
2 teaspoons butter or Extra Virgin Olive Oil

-in a saucepan add water, Better Than Bouillon, Parsley, Butter and bring to a rapid boil
-add Rice and cook according to directions

Red Rice

1 cup brown Basmati Rice
2 cups Water
2 Tablespoons tomato paste or 1 cup of crushed Tomato Sauce
½ Tablespoon Vege-Sal
½ onion Chopped
1 Celery rib chopped
½ Green Pepper chopped

-add all ingredients except Rice to water
-when water boils add rice and follow directions

Cornbread

In our home, there is nothing that screams home made like hot skillet Cornbread. It is an excellent accompaniment to absolutely everything and if my husband had his way he would eat it every day! Here are two variations on making Cornbread. This is truly Southern Comfort on a plate.

2 cups Yellow Cornmeal
4 teaspoons Aluminum Free Baking Powder
5 Tablespoons Organic Cane Sugar
½ teaspoon Salt
1 Egg beaten
1 cup Milk
2 Tablespoons Extra Virgin Olive Oil

-place a greased cast iron skillet in the oven on 425
-mix all ingredients in a bowl until mixed but not too smooth
-once skillet is hot, remove and pour in corn mix
-cook at least 20 minutes until golden brown cut like a pie and cut pats of butter on top

Hot Water Cornbread

2 cups Yellow Cornmeal
1 cup boiling hot Water
1 Egg
¼ teaspoon Parsley
¼ teaspoon Vege-Sal
Pinch of Organic Cane Sugar
Extra Virgin Olive Oil

-mix all ingredients together except hot Water in a mixing bowl
-heat oil in skillet
-add boiling hot Water to bowl
-mix together well
-scoop 1 Tablespoon of mix into hot Oil, cook until brown and then flip
-serve immediately with Butter

Mozzarella Cheesy Garlic Bread

1 loaf fresh baked Multi-Grain French Bread
6 Tablespoons Garlic minced super fine
1 stick melted Butter
1 ball fresh Mozzarella Cheese

-slice French Bread on the side to open

-brush on melted Butter
-load on minced Garlic
-cover bread with Mozzarella Cheese
-bake in oven on 450 until bubbly and browned around the edges

Cranberry Sauce

Once this homemade version of Cranberry Sauce hit my table the old canned version was history.

1 package fresh whole cranberries
¾ cup organic cane sugar
1 cup water
1 Orange fresh squeezed juice
1 Tablespoon Orange Zest

-wash Cranberries and pick out the bruised
-in a pot boil Water and sugar until reaches boiling
-add in Cranberries and let them boil stirring constantly– they will pop open like popcorn
-stir in fresh Orange Juice and Orange Zest
-pour all contents into a glass bowl – allow to cool
-cover bowl and refrigerate until jells like jell o
-serve on Dressing or on the side of the plate
* TIP – buy cranberries when in season and freeze in freezer bags to have all year long. Keep on hand to add into muffins, cakes, salads.

Nutritional Note:
Cranberries are loaded with fiber to help alleviate constipation and other bowel dysfunctions. They also contain a super-dose of Vitamin C. For the Cranberry Juice enthusiast consider making fresh Cranberry Juice instead of the store varieties that contain too much sugar. Your body will thank you.

Fried Green Tomatoes

During the Tomato growing season, most farmers will reserve a quantity of Green Tomatoes for customers like me who love to have them Fried, as Salsa, or Salsa Verde. Here are some variations:

2 Green Tomatoes
1 Egg beaten
1 cup Organic Corn Meal
1 teaspoon Himalayan Salt
1 teaspoon Garlic Powder
1 teaspoon Onion Powder
1/2 teaspoon Cayenne Pepper
1/2 cup Extra Virgin Olive Oil or Grape Seed Oil

-wash and dry the Green Tomato and slice between the two navels revealing the chamber-like cross-section
-slice into 1/2 inch slices
-heat a cast iron skillet on medium heat with just enough oil to cover the bottom of the pan

Kitchen Warriors 101: Homemade Healthy

-beat Egg into 1 bowl with a Tablespoon of water (this is called Egg Wash, the water helps adherence of the Cornmeal)
-in a mixing bowl add all dry ingredients and blend well
-dip front and back of sliced Tomato in the Egg wash and then dredge it in the seasoned Cornmeal
-place in the hot oil and watch the edges turn brown before turning only once
-drain on a paper towel and serve immediately

TIP: I do not use flour because all of the powdered substances are flour-like and mixing them with the Cornmeal also helps adherence.

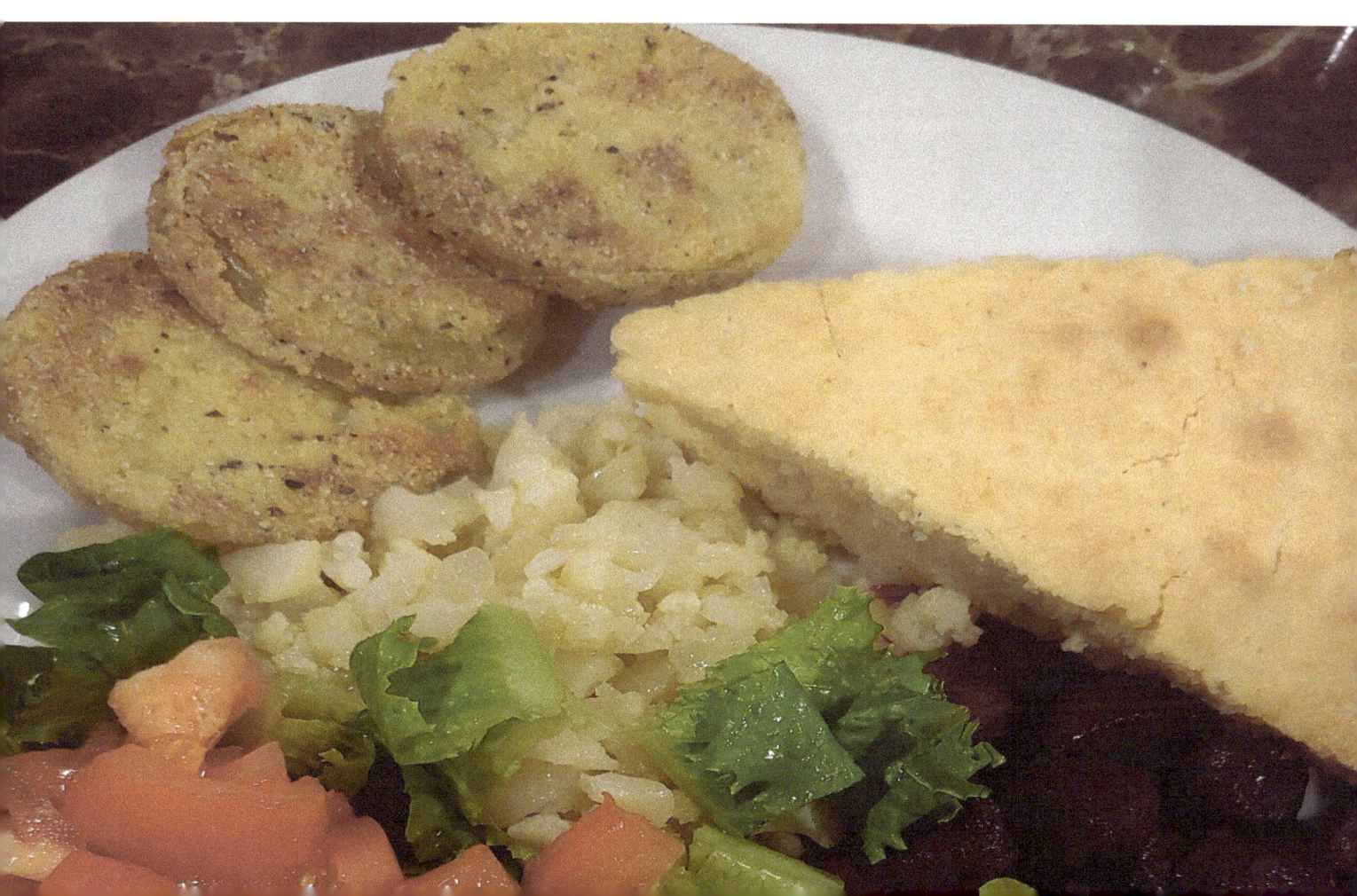

Salsa Verde

4 Green Tomatoes
1 White Onion
1 Habanero Pepper (optional)
2 Garlic Cloves
2 Tablespoons Cumin
3-4 springs Cilantro
1 teaspoon Himalayan Salt
1 cup Water

-chop and place all ingredients in a medium sized soup pot with Water
-cook low and slow until all is practically a soup
-allow to cool and blend a little at a time until all is done
-warm when ready to serve and put on top of chicken, fish or vegetables

Beets

1 bunch of fresh Beets with the Tops
1 small yellow onion chopped
1 Tablespoon Bragg's Apple Cider Vinegar with The Mother
1 Teaspoon Organic Brown Sugar
1 Tablespoon Butter
1 Four Quart Saucepan

-thoroughly wash all grit off of the Beets and Tops
-peel the skin off of the Beets and chop into 1/4 inch cubes

- in Saucepan add Beet cubes, Onions and Apple Cider Vinegar with enough water to cover them
- cook covered on low until Beets are almost fork-tender then add Brown Sugar and chopped Tops
- when Beets have reached desired tenderness, add Butter and stir

Nutritional Note:
Beets are high in Manganese which helps to protect cells from damage, strong bones, blood clotting, and strong immunity. They are high in Iron, Folate, Vitamin C, and Potassium too. Juicing Beets or eating them in conjunction with Spinach packs a powerful punch when Iron in the body is low. Additionally, Beets have been reported to stimulate blood flow, which men deem as important.

Cauliflower Rice

With the Paleo craze has come a bevvy of uses for un-popular vegetables and Cauliflower is one of them which will substitute rice and grains easily. Cauliflower is one of the vegetables which can take on the taste of whatever you decide. This is just one of the many variations and worth a try not just because Paleo is now your thing, but because it is delicious.

1 head of Cauliflower cleaned and cored
1/4 oil of choice
1 large Onion chopped
1 teaspoon Vege-Sal
1 teaspoon Garlic Powder

1 teaspoon Onion Powder
1 Soup Pot

-after cleaning Cauliflower, break into chunks to ensure it is dry
-use a food processor to chop but not liquefy (I prefer to chop by hand on a cutting board and it takes less time than wrangling with the food processor set-up and clean-up.)
-in a large Soup Pot put Oil, chopped Onions, Garlic Powder, Onion Powder and Vege-Sal and allow it to sautee together until onions are clear
-add the chopped Cauliflower and toss to coat all of the ingredients
-add about 1/2 cup of water toss again and cover until desired tenderness is reached

TIP:
Add absolutely any flavor along with a protein of choice or enjoy like Fried Rice.

Nutritional Note:
Cauliflower is a cruciferous vegetable and has 100% of the daily recommended amount of Vitamin C, is high in Fiber, and an excellent source of Antioxidants. It is very low in Carbohydrates which is why it is favorable for those embarking on the Paleo Lifestyle.

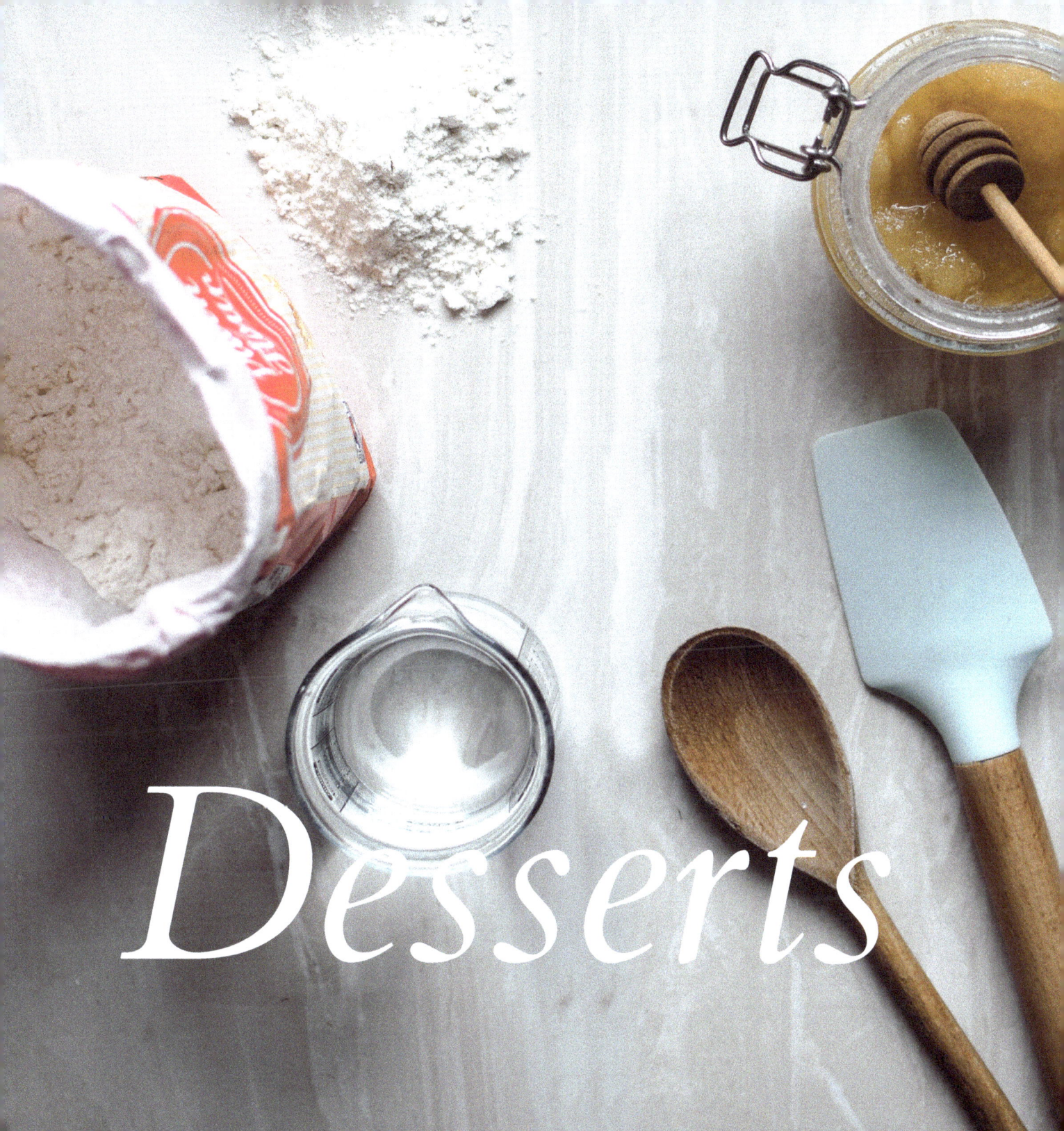

I cannot stress enough that the ingredients used for baking make all of the difference in the world to the taste. Organic Unbleached Flour, Sea Salt, organic Extracts, organic Sugar will gain great results. My one secret weapon is the type of Vanilla Extract used…Vanilla Extracto from a Hispanic country. The Vanilla Extracto from Puerto Rico, Dominican Republic, Mexico is simply ooooohh la la. It is darker, richer, more concentrated, and tastier than most popular brands, and…while it is not listed as organic, there is not vast listing of ingredients that are difficult to pronounce. Venture into a Hispanic neighborhood grocery store or make a purchase on an island while traveling. It is worth the effort.

Grannie and LaJoyce's Signature Coconut Cake

When my Grannie made this cake you could taste the love she put into it. She would literally whip the batter by hand all day. The batter would sit in a bowl and every time she passed it, she would whip it 100 strokes or more. By the time the cake was baked it was the lightest, and fluffy-ist cake to ever cross your lips.

4 cups sifted Organic Unbleached Flour
2 sticks Butter softened at room temperature
1 cup Sugar
4 Eggs room temperature
2 teaspoons Aluminum Free Baking Powder
2 Tablespoons Vanilla
1 teaspoon Lemon
1 cup Milk room temperature
1 bag Coconut
1 jar Pineapple Preserves
1 box Organic Vanilla Frosting or 1 can Vanilla Frosting

-sift the Flour 3-4 times
-cream Sugar and Butter by hand
-add all other ingredients one by one by hand until well blended
-using mixer blend on high
-bake for 30-35 minutes at 350 in greased and floured baking pans
-remove cakes from pans and place on cooling rack

-place 1 cake layer face down onto cake dish and spread Pineapple Preserves on thickly
-put the other cake layer on top - bottom side down
-gently spread frosting all over tops and sides of cake
-liberally apply coconut to sides and top ensuring it sticks
*WARNING…don't hurt yourself

Chicago "Lunch Room" Butter Cookies

Anyone who went to Chicago Public Schools from the 1960s-1980s was a lover of these cookies when we were kids. Since my mother was a teacher, she made friends with the lunchroom lady who gave us this recipe. I re-wrote the recipe from the raggedy original on a snowy day and that notebook paper re-write is dated December 10, 1977. I keep it in a Ziploc bag to protect it and have substituted all of the ingredients to organic to heighten their flavor. I give out these cookies along with my Eggnog every Christmas to the people around town and my neighbors. I also mail the cookies to relatives and friends. My good friend Terri has found a way to savor them for months by putting the cookies in the freezer and eating them as a cool treat. Homemade goodies go a really long way and show a deep and sincere appreciation that the time was taken to prepare items just for them.

1 pound Butter at room temperature
4 cups unbleached Flour sifted
2 cups Powdered Sugar
1 ½ Tablespoon Vanilla
A pinch Sea Salt

-sift Flour into a bowl
-in a large bowl cream Butter and Sugar by hand with a wooden spoon
-add Salt and Extract
-mix in one cup of Flour at a time

Kitchen Warriors 101: Homemade Healthy

-scoop 1 heaping teaspoon of cookie dough into hand and roll into a ball
-place balls on a cookie sheet 1 inch apart and press down flat with two fingers to leave an imprint in the cookie round
-cook for about 6 minutes at 400 until light brown

Lemon extract
Vanilla extract
Pinch ginger
½ can Pet Milk or Evaporated Milk
1 Pie Crust

-wash and boil the Sweet Potatoes in the skin
-when fork tender, drain and allow to cool completely before handling
-peel skin and mash Sweet Potatoes in a bowl
-mash Sweet Potatoes in a bowl
-add all ingredients one at a time
-check for taste and add accordingly
-bake until golden brown on 350

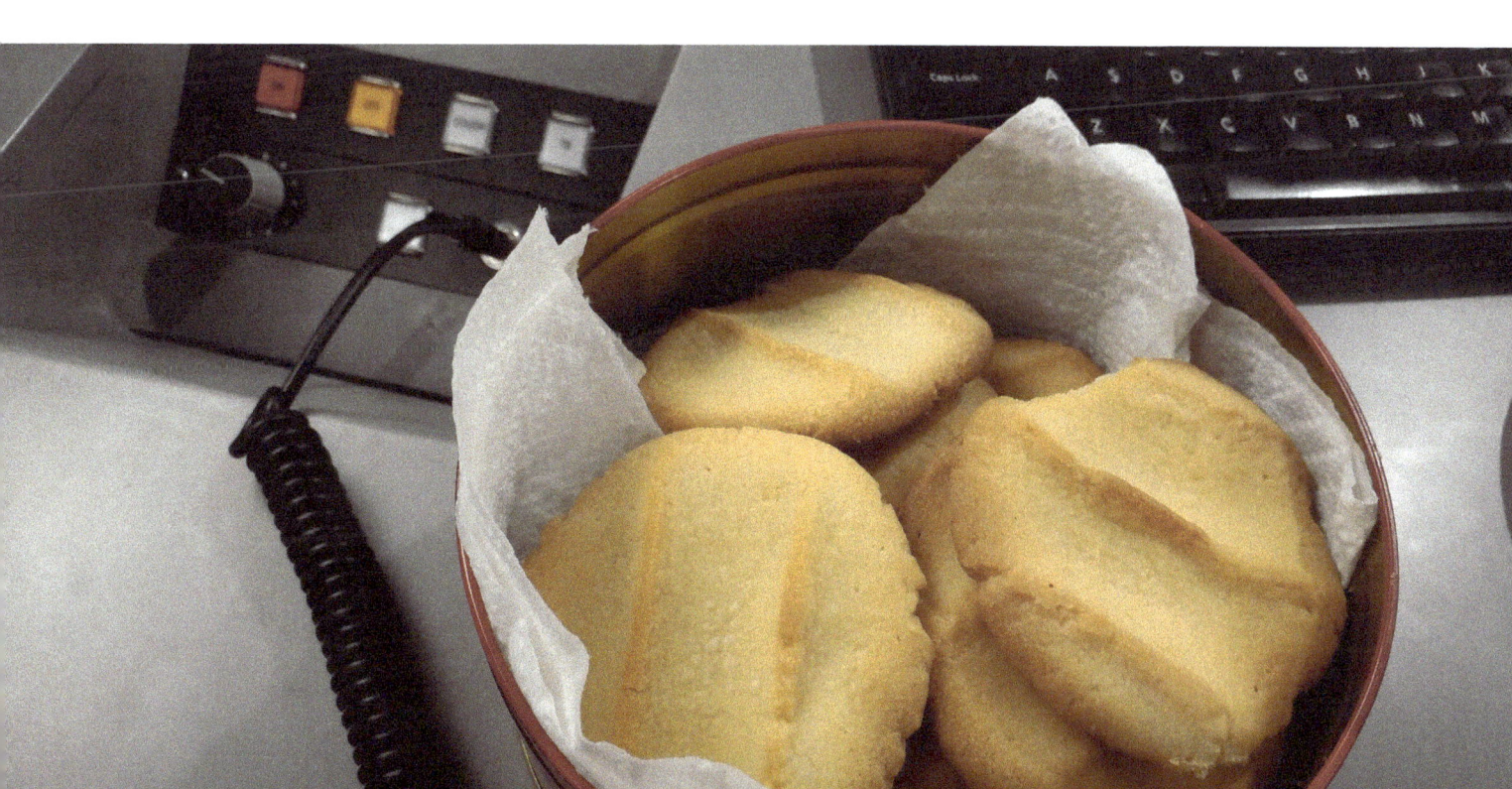

Dr. LaJoyce Brookshire

Gus' Oh My Apple Pie

I may cook everything in my house but it is my husband Gus who makes the Apple Pie *Oh, my...*

1 bag of Organic Red Delicious Apples cored, skinned, cubed
2 Pie Crusts cut in strips
2 sticks Butter
½ cup Cinnamon
1 ½ cup Sugar
½ cup Red Bob Mills Pancake Mix
2 cups Water
Large baking dish

- cut Apples into a bowl and toss with Cinnamon, Sugar and Pancake Mix
- place Apples in a greased baking dish – pour water on top of Apples – place teaspoons of Butter all around the chopped Apples
- arrange Pie Crust strips lattice style on top of the Apples with Butter and sprinkle Cinnamon and Sugar liberally
- pour Water into the dish until it is half-way to the top
- bake at 350 until Apples are tender, Water begins to bubble, and top is golden brown
*WARNING – Having this dessert around could be habit forming.

Nutritional Note:
Apples are very high in antioxidants and flavonoids and rich in Vitamin C and Potassium. Reserve the Apple skins in a BPA-Free Ziploc bag for Smoothies. Apples are very heavily pesticided so be sure to always purchase organic. The skins have a great deal of minerals and fiber. An Apple a day really does keep the doctor away.

Mama Brookshire's Sweet Potato Pie

When Gus Brookshire learned how to make an Apple Pie it was definitely from Mama Brookshire, because my Mom-In-Law can burn! Her Sweet Potato Pies are the most requested item at the Mt. Moriah Missionary Baptist Church in Chicago, True Light Baptist Church in Walnut Grove, Mississippi, and from anyone else who has ever had a sliver. Part of the deliciousness is that she never measures a thing. "I just go with it the flavors," she always says. I have to admit, sometimes I can hit it like Mama, and sometimes I completely miss. Good luck!...

2 pounds Sweet Potatoes boiled and skinned
¾ cup Organic Cane Sugar
2 Eggs
1 stick Butter softened
Nutmeg
Cinnamon
Lemon extract
Vanilla extract
Pinch ginger
½ can Pet Milk or Evaporated Milk
1 Pie Crust
-mash Sweet Potatoes in a bowl
-add all ingredients one at a time
-check for taste and add accordingly
-bake until golden brown on 350

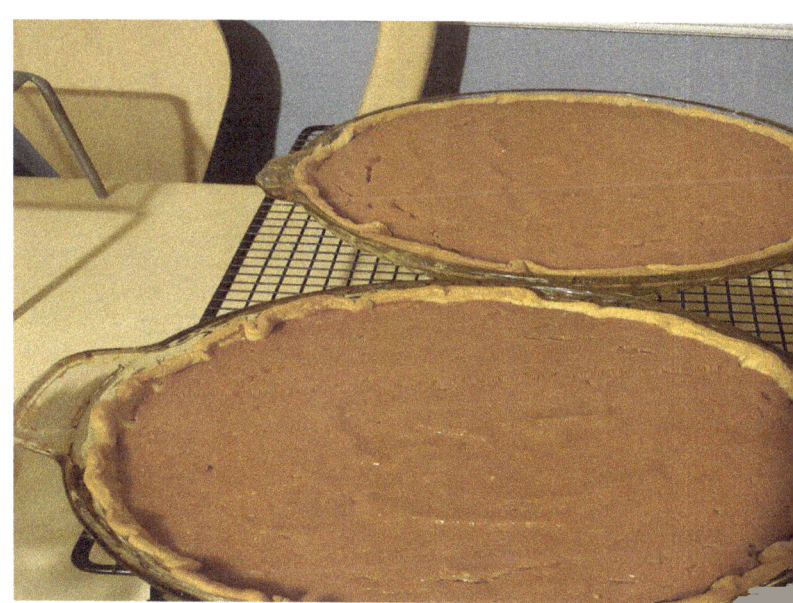

desserts

Pineapple Upside Down Cake

My Aunt Anita was the family master at making a Rich Golden Cake batter. It tastes better than any 1-2-3-4 cake you have ever tasted. In 2009 on a weekend visit to her home she gifted me with the hand-written recipe card file that was curated by my Great-Grandmother. From it I learned the cake baking trick… this batter is the beginning for ANY cake she makes and adding the pineapples is a sweet surprise! I have substituted the recipe for healthier options and cut way back on the sugar. To make a larger cake double everything listed including the cooking time.

2 ¼ cups sifted Unbleached Flour
1 ½ cups Organic Cane Sugar
1-2 cups of Organic Brown Sugar (Light or Dark)
3 teaspoons Aluminum-Free Baking Powder
1 teaspoon Salt
2/3 cup soft Organic Shortening or Butter
1 cup Organic Milk
1 ½ Tablespoon Vanilla
3 Organic Eggs (room temperature)
-1-2 cans of Crushed Pineapples

-drain Crushed Pineapples pressing out juice into a bowl (save liquid for a Coco Colada)
-liberally grease an oblong baking pan
-shake brown sugar on the bottom of the pan until covered
-hand press the sugar into base of the pan until smooth with no clumps
-spoon the drained Crushed Pineapples on top of the Brown Sugar and gently spread around evenly

Kitchen Warriors 101: Homemade Healthy

-In a mixing bowl: cream Butter or Shortening, Organic Cane Sugar, and Vanilla together until smooth
-add Eggs one at a time
-sift together Flour, Baking Powder, and Salt and add to the mixing bowl a little at a time
-slowly pour-in Milk last
-pour completed mix on top of the Pineapples and bake at 350 degrees for 45 minutes or until a toothpick comes out clean
-allow cake to cool-off for about 10 minutes then using a spatulas, gently release the cake around the edges
-to turn the cake upside down, place an oblong cake tray atop of the pan
-using hand mitts, turn the cake upside down.
-BEFORE removing the oblong baking pan, tap the bottom of the pan to release anything that may be stuck and then remove the pan to reveal the masterpiece! Allow to cool a bit before serving.

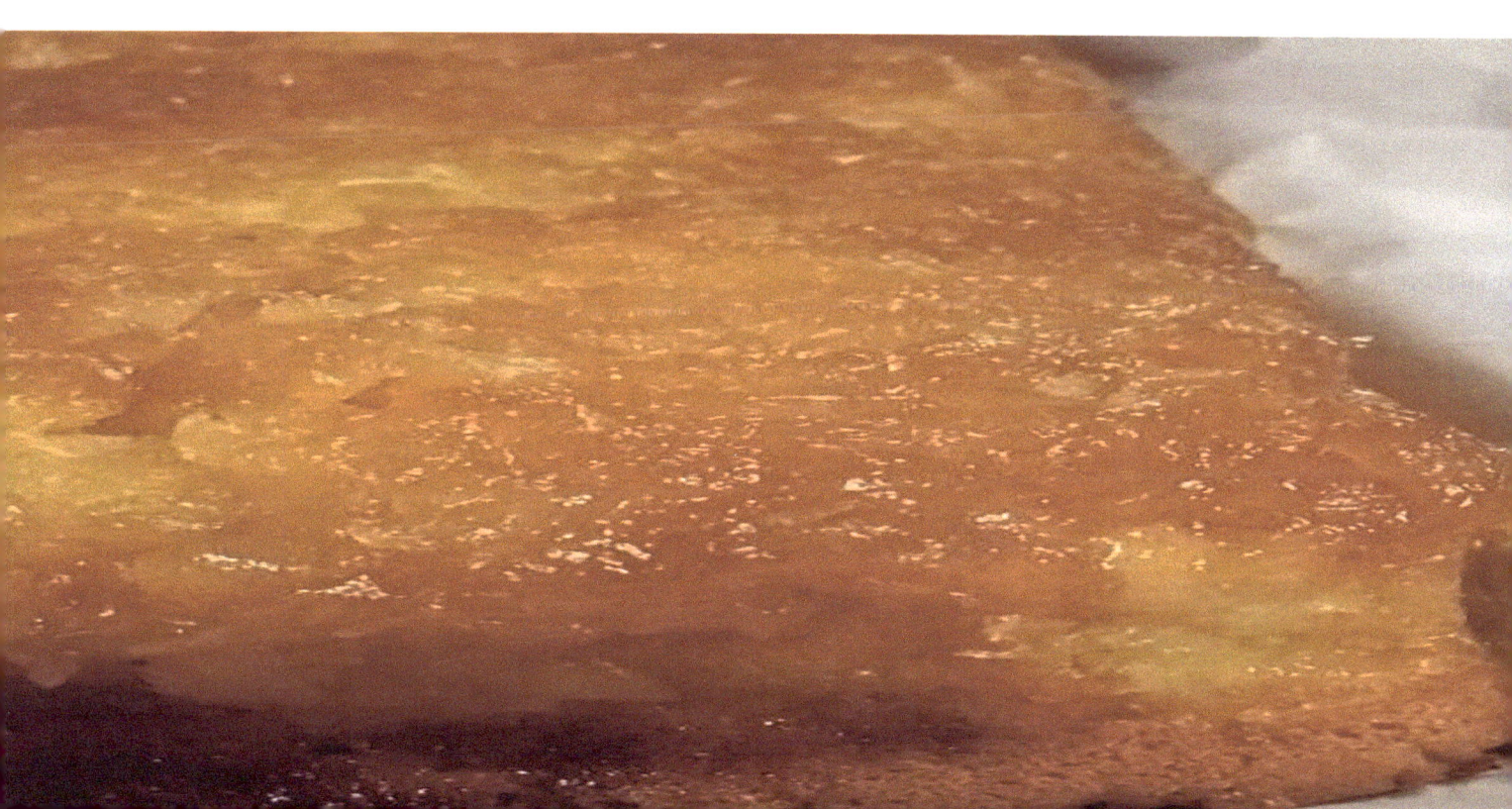

Biscotti

My beloved high school Spanish and home room teacher Susan Pauletti and I discovered our love for home baked goodies back when I was just a freshman in 1976. We have remained in close contact through the years and during my annual visit to her home we bake her wonderful Biscotti to have with a cup of tea.

1 ½ sticks Butter
1 ½ cups Organic Cane Sugar
2 Tablespoons Vanilla Extract
1 Tablespoon Almond Extract
4 Eggs beaten
4 cups unbleached Flour sifted
4 teaspoons aluminum free Baking Powder
1 cup Almonds, Walnuts, or Pecans chopped
Powdered Sugar (optional)
1 bag Dark Chocolate bits (optional)-cream Butter and Sugar with a wooden spoon
-add Eggs slowly plus Extract
-mix in 1 cup of Flour at a time
-blend in Nuts last
-roll dough into a ball and cut in half
-roll out each half onto a cookie sheet into a snake roll
-cut the dough on an angle at least 1 ½ inch long
-bake at 350 until brown
-shake powdered sugar over the Biscotti when done
-or-
-instead of Nuts add Dark Chocolate bits
-or-

-use Nuts and put the Dark Chocolate bits on the outside to melt and smear
*TIP – This is yummy any way you create it. Will keep in a covered container about 1 week.

Bundt Cake a La Maureen

My neighbor Maureen has mastered how to bake with only fruit and no sugar. I am a work in progress in this effort as it is still hit or miss as she does not measure quantities. Each time I watch her it is different. I am getting close to her perfection with the quantities below. I would love to hear about your results!

3 Bananas ripened and mashed
1 1/2 cups Blueberries (or any fruit)
3 Eggs
1 stick Butter melted
1 ½ cups Organic Coffee Creamer or Coconut Creamer by So Delicious
3 Tablespoons Vanilla
4 cups organic unbleached Flour sifted

-pre-heat oven to 350
-Butter Bundt pan
-blend Bananas until smooth
-add all flour to Bananas
-fold in all liquid ingredients
-batter should drip from the mixer, add more Creamer until drips freely
-fold in fruit gently
-bake for about 1 hour until toothpick comes out clean

desserts

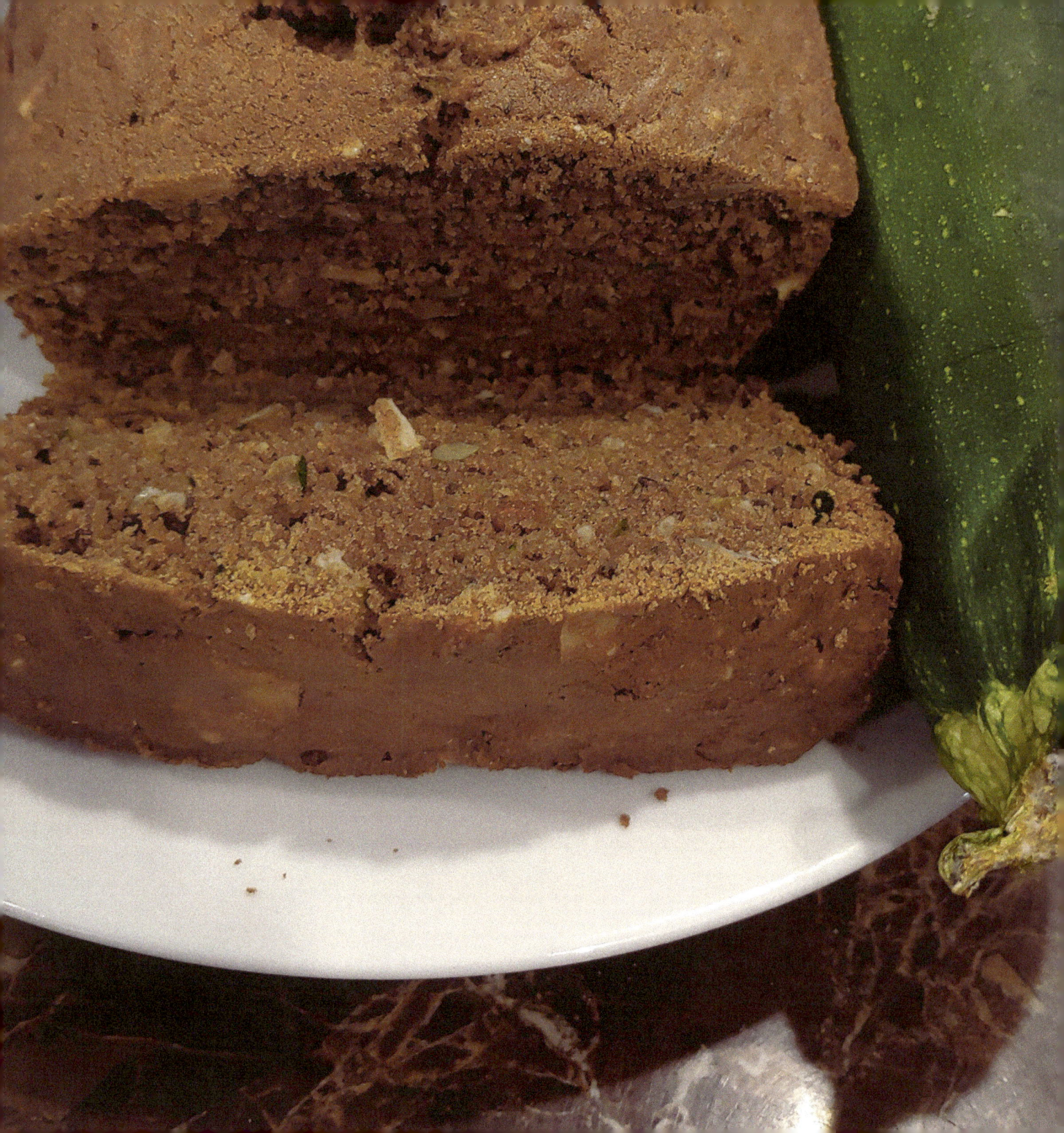

Zucchini Bread

As a member of a Community Shared Garden, when Zucchini season is in full-swing I have had to become creative on what to do with all of the loot. This Zucchini Bread recipe is a winner for breakfast, lunch, dinner or an anytime snack. Most of the recipes I had found have too much sugar for it to be healthy so I have finagled this recipe until it is what I believe to be perfection! My family loves the guilt-free indulgence and my SiriusXM Team loves when I bring Zucchini Bread to the studio. It also freezes well when wrapped in freezer paper and a BPA-Free Freezer Storage Bag.

3/4 cup roughly chopped Walnuts or Pecans Optional
3/4 cup melted Coconut Oil
-or-
1/2 cup Extra Virgin Olive Oil
1/2 cup Honey or Maple Syrup
1/2 cup Organic Milk of choice or Water
1 teaspoon Baking Soda
1 teaspoon Cinnamon + more to add to the top
2 teaspoons Vanilla Extract
1/2 teaspoon fine grain Sea Salt
1/4 teaspoon ground Nutmeg
1 1/2 cups grated Zucchini (1 small or medium)
1 3/4 cups Whole Wheat Flour

It is best to plan to bake this bread as all ingredients should be room temperature:
-grate Zucchini and wring-out excess water in paper towels

Dr. LaJoyce Brookshire

Aunt Mabel's Perfected Cinnamon Rolls

This recipe is our family favorite! When we were kids, Aunt Mabel would give us these rolls hot out of the oven with a glass of milk and we would be in Heaven. In November 2008, I drove four hours to Riverhead Long Island to Aunt Mabel's house because she personally invited to teach me how to make the Yeast Rolls and the Cinnamon Rolls before she forgot. Please understand…this is a huge project. It takes Gus, Brooke, and me to get the job done. The reward is simply indescribable.

It takes Gus, Brooke, and me to get the job done. The reward is simply indescribable. I am the only one in our family who has learned from the master on how to make them. It is now my responsibility to supply the family with the rolls on demand. I got the stamp of approval on my revisions from Aunt Anita when she called to say, "Girl, what in the world did you do to these rolls? You ought to be arrested!"

Dough – (Makes 50 Buns)
3 cups Milk scalded
2/3 cup Organic Shortening
2/3 cup Organic Cane Sugar
1 ½ Tablespoons Sea Salt
1 ½ oz fresh Cake Yeast room temperature
(buy a block of yeast from a baker, slice into 2 oz slices, and freeze – can last 4 months in freezer – thaw by placing in fridge or on counter)
3 medium organic Eggs room temperature
9 ½ cups sifted unbleached Flour
1 pound Butter

desserts

Cinnamon Mix
1 cup Cinnamon
2 cups Organic Cane Sugar
1 ½ cup Chopped Pecans or Walnuts
1 20oz can Organic Raisins

Frosting
2 packages organic Powdered Sugar
1 stick Butter
1 cup Half & Half (or more for thinner texture)
4 Tablespoons Vanilla
A food Thermometer
-sift Flour saving 4 ounces separately
-in a saucepan scald Milk then add Shortening, Sugar, and Salt stirring until blended
-cool until warm at 120 degrees
-crumble Yeast into mix and stir blending Eggs well
-add liquid to sifted Flour kneading in the 4 ounces of Flour
-liberally grease a bowl with a handful of Shortening, place dough in the bowl, grease the top of the dough with a thin layer of Butter, cover with a clean towel and let rise in a warm place for about 2 hours
-grease fist with Shortening and punch down dough in the center
-cover again and let rise for 20 minutes
-chop Nuts and mix Cinnamon and Sugar into a bowl or a shake out container
-Flour counter or table and roll out dough with a rolling pin
-smear butter thickly over the rolled-out dough
-cut the dough in half

MUST WORK QUICKLY AS DOUGH BEGINS TO RISE:
-liberally shake the Cinnamon Sugar mix over the Butter covering every spot
-cover Cinnamon Sugar with Raisins

Dr. LaJoyce Brookshire

-cover Raisins with Nuts
-roll both halves of dough the long way into a tight log-roll
-sprinkle the top of the log-rolls with the cinnamon-sugar mix
-cut in to 1 inch slices and place 6 in a row in a greased pan
-cover with a towel and put in a warm place to rise again
(This step is not necessary but it sure adds to the fluffy!)

Make frosting while rolls are rising:
-mix Butter and Powdered Sugar together
-slowly add-in Half & Half
-add Vanilla until frosting turns light brown – the more Vanilla the more intense the flavor –
the more intense the frosting the yummier!
-let frosting stand at room temp

-bake rolls at 350 until browned about 30 minutes or more
-remove from oven and spoon frosting on top

* WARNING – Arrest warrants **will** be pending.

I pray that these recipes will help to enhance your Wellness Journey. When meal planning, select an item from each category: Beverages, Entrées, Vegetables, and Desserts. It is my hope this takes out the guess-work about what to prepare for healthy meals.

I encourage you to vary these recipes to *your* liking. Just remember, You Are What You Eat, so go easy on the greasy☺. Foods are meant to be enjoyed. Foods can heal and a good meal can heal both the body and the soul.

As you try these dishes incorporate them into your week for a healthy variation and watch your health improve along the way.

I want to hear from you. Let me know how you enjoyed the dishes. Ultimately I want to hear your health Praise Reports because your perfect health is good food for my soul.

ASK THE GOOD DOCTOR

Thank You

I wish to thank my Heavenly Father from whom all blessings flow. God has continually blessed me with the gift to create delicious and nutritious meals so that we can have the stamina to spread the Gospel.

I wish to thank the following people who have made an indelible mark upon my Wellness Journey:

My Bo Daddy…He was my first Royal Taste-Tester! No matter the time of day, if we saw something on TV that looked good to eat he would say, "I'll go buy it if you make it." I made many blunders and created many masterpieces through the years and he was always there as my champion to try again. Thank you for shining your light from Heaven and I hope I have made you proud.

My Husband Gus…You continue to challenge me by calling every day around 3:30pm asking the Question of the Day, "What's for Dinner?" I can count on you to make this phone call and my response determines whether or not you grab a snack. The desire to keep you healthy inspires me to keep something yummy cooking in the kitchen that brings you right to the dinner table. Who loves you bay-ba?

My Angel Girl Brooke…You are always ready for something tasty. I am so delighted that you have such an expansive palette. Thank you for trying anything I will place in front of you at least once. I have come to respect your opinion about the "Yuck" and the "Yummy" and I enjoy eating your creations as you have learned well. Mommy loves you!

My Publisher Elissa Gabrielle…You are an amazing visionary! Thank you for pushing me in this direction and out of my comfort zone. You have spoken this project to life and I appreciate you. We are making Mama Mike proud of us!

My Book Cover and Interior Designer Jessica Tilles…Thank you for taking Elissa's cover vision and bringing to fruition a lovely work of art! And for converting my mess and making a masterpiece. I appreciate your skills greatly. Let's do it again soon.

My Photographer Elijah (Farmer) Muhammad for EMPhotography…You are such an awesome photographer, hence the nickname "One-Shot-Johnny"! I truly appreciate your perfection, your professionalism, and your friendship. We have been through thick and thin and we are still standing!

My Sister Friend Debra Fraser-Howze…When I asked if we could use your kitchen for this cover shoot, you said, "YES" without hesitation! Thank you for allowing us to ascend upon your home with a full crew, food, flood lights, and barrels of laughter. I am eternally grateful for how you continually show yourself to me not just a friend, but as family.

Thank you to my awesome SiriusXM Team Irvin Wright, Michelle Joyce, Alexa Zaromatidis, Tremell McKenzie, and Karen Hunter for bringing the ASK THE GOOD DOCTOR vision to fruition!

www.ingramcontent.com/pod-product-compliance
Lightning Source LLC
LaVergne TN
LVHW071953290426
837647LV00030B/2741